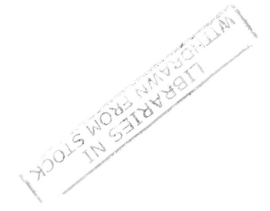

The
ALLERGY-FREE
FAMILY
COOKBOOK

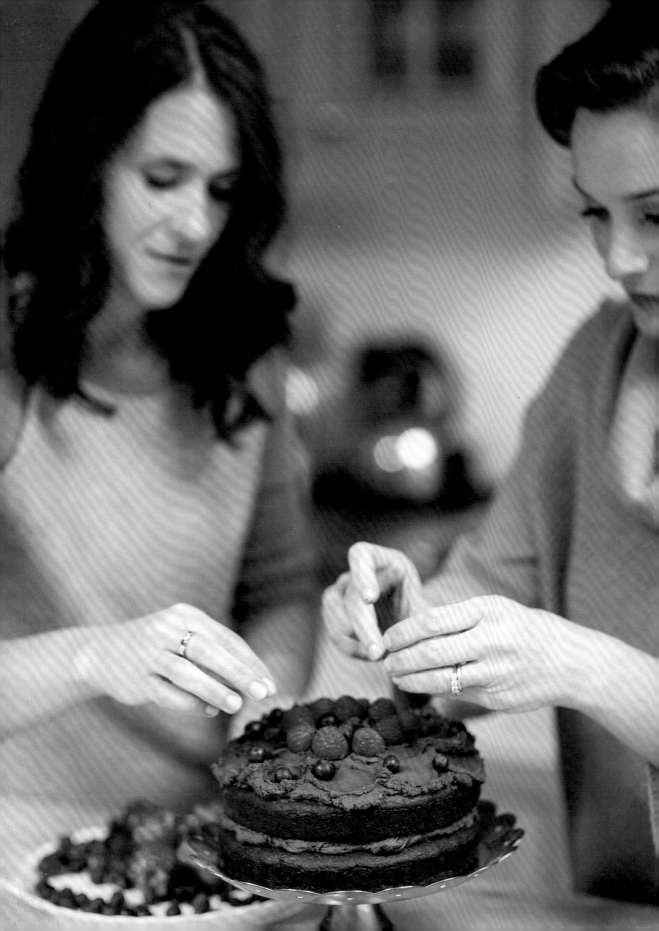

The

ALLERGY-FREE
FAMILY
COOKBOOK

Fiona Heggie & Ellie Lux

First published in Great Britain in 2015
by Orion Publishing Group Ltd
Carmelite House, 50 Victoria Embankment
London EC4Y 0DZ
An Hachette UK Company

10 9 8 7 6 5 4 3

A CIP catalogue record for this book is available from the British Library.

ISBN: 978 1 4091 5581 2

Photography by Chris Terry
Design by Smith & Gilmour
Illustrations by Debbie Powell
Props by Olivia Wardle
Food styling by Henrietta Clancy
Edited by Abi Waters
Proofread by Jennifer Wheatley
Indexed by Elizabeth Wiggans

Printed and bound in China

The Orion Publishing Group's policy is to use papers that are
natural, renewable and recyclable products and made from wood
grown in sustainable forests. The logging and manufacturing
processes are expected to conform to the environmental
regulations of the country of origin.

www.orionbooks.co.uk

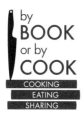

For lots more delicious recipes plus articles, interviews
and videos from the best chefs cooking today visit our blog
bybookorbycook.co.uk

Follow us

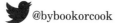 @bybookorcook

Find us

 facebook.com/bybookorbycook

CONTENTS

Introduction

It's daunting when your child is diagnosed with a food allergy. You immediately focus on the negatives: the foods they can't eat, the meals they won't get to enjoy, the nutrients that will be missing from their diets and the hassle involved in adapting recipes, eating out and checking food labels.

This book is about the positives. Just because your child is allergic to one – or, indeed, several – foods doesn't mean that they can't eat delicious meals with the rest of the family and benefit from a balanced diet or nice treats – should they deserve them! The truth is that there is an almost endless range of meals that you can cook for your children using ordinary ingredients readily found in every supermarket.

It is also worth remembering that you're not alone. Allergies are on the increase with 6 percent of children now being diagnosed as allergic to one or multiple foods. That includes our children. And yet, when Isabelle and Casper were diagnosed with multiple food allergies, we found that there was surprisingly little practical advice out there or cookbooks that catered for multiple food allergies.

WHERE IT ALL STARTED

Ellie's daughter, Isabelle, had severe eczema as a baby and still suffers with asthma, which has resulted in numerous hospital stays. When she first ate a piece of cheese, Isabelle immediately came out in hives all over her body and face and both her eyes puffed and closed up – she was quite clearly allergic to dairy. She subsequently tested positive for immediate allergies to egg, sesame and peanut (from which she is at significant risk of anaphylactic shock). Isabelle also gets hayfever and is allergic to dogs and house dust mites. She has, in other words, what the doctors refer to as a very typical (if quite severe) atopic profile.

Fiona's son Casper has an immediate allergy to egg, which was discovered in testing when he had severe eczema and was clearly a problem when he ate some cake and reacted immediately. As with Izzy, subsequent testing showed he also had an immediate allergy to peanuts. In addition, Casper has delayed allergy to gluten, which caused him severe gastrointestinal problems. And there was a time when he couldn't eat dairy or soya either as he had to eliminate these foods in order to help determine which allergen was causing the problems. He is one of the increasing number of children who have a combination of immediate and delayed food allergies, which meant his diagnosis was less straightforward than Isabelle's but the management of both types is the same: avoid the food allergens causing the problems.

We would, of course, rather that our children weren't allergic to anything. There have been scares, frustrations and inconveniences. But in the grand scheme of things, they have been minor.

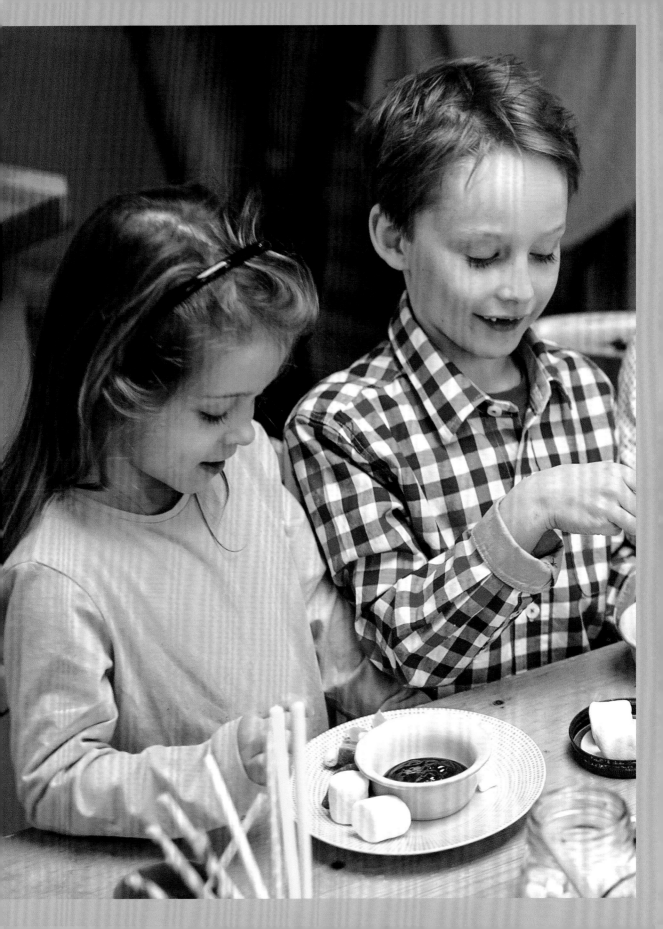

ENDORSED BY EXPERTS

We have both been lucky to have had wonderful support from doctors and dietitians. Dr Helen Cox is one of just a handful of paediatric consultants specialising in allergy and immunology. Dr Rosan Meyer is a leading dietitian focusing on food allergy in children. They both run clinics where they see hundreds of children with food allergies every year and we are very grateful to them for lending their expertise in reviewing and endorsing this book.

OUR FRIENDSHIP

We have been friends since we were 11-years-old and our two families spend a lot of time together. We often compared notes about cooking healthy food for our kids (preferably without slaving for hours in the kitchen to produce it). If either of us was cooking a meal that Isabelle and Casper were both eating, it had to be free from five different food allergens. It was over one of those meals that we came up with the idea for this book.

Fiona has always been passionate about food; she trained at Leith's School of Food and Wine in London and has run a successful catering business. Before Isabelle was born Ellie could barely boil an egg. Fiona was the brains behind most of the recipes, but if Ellie couldn't cook them they didn't make it into the book.

The result is a collection of over 100 recipes that are delicious, healthy, quick and easy to cook, and can be enjoyed by your whole family. All the recipes just happen to be free of eight common allergens: dairy, eggs, peanuts, tree nuts, soya, gluten, sesame and shellfish.

ADJUSTING THE RECIPES

We are conscious that most children won't be allergic to all eight allergens; more likely it'll be a combination of a few or a couple of them. So we've explained how you can add back the ingredients to which your child is not allergic – there's no point eliminating foods unnecessarily when your child's diet is already restricted.

MAKING LIFE EASY

We are busy parents and know it's crucial that feeding your child fits easily into the rest of your life. We both have younger children, Camille and Zara, who have no allergies, but they always eat the same meals as their older siblings. We've arranged our recipes into categories we found helpful and that reflect how we cook for our children. Your whole family can enjoy these meals and there's no need to cater separately for your allergic child or for them to feel they're being treated differently or missing out.

ADVICE AND TIPS

But this is more than just a cookbook. Food allergy clearly needs to be taken seriously, but it does not have to change your life – with the right advice it can actually be straightforward to manage.

So in this book we've also shared what we've learned from our experience in managing food allergy.

We hope that the result is more than just a cookery book with wholesome, tasty family recipes using ordinary ingredients; it is also a handbook that any parent can rely on and refer to for accurate information and advice on every practical aspect of dealing with their children's food allergies.

FOOD ALLERGY
Explained by Dr Helen Cox

Dr Helen Cox is a leading expert in her field – paediatric allergy and immunology – and has extensive experience in the management of children with food allergy. She is one of the clinical lead consultants in paediatric allergy at Imperial College Healthcare NHS.

If your son or daughter is one of the six percent of children in the UK diagnosed with a food allergy then you are bound to have questions. Let's start with the most difficult one first.

WHY IS FOOD ALLERGY ON THE INCREASE?

There has been plenty of research into food allergy but, disappointingly, much of it has yielded conflicting results.

The lower rates of eczema, food allergy, asthma and allergic rhinitis in Third World countries lead experts to believe that the increase in allergies could be down to relatively recent changes in developed world lifestyles. There are a variety of theories that focus on genetics, epigenetics (the study of how genes can in some circumstances be altered by external factors), the environment, diet and infections.

But the frustrating answer is that we still don't know.

WHAT IS THE DIFFERENCE BETWEEN FOOD HYPERSENSITIVITY, FOOD INTOLERANCE AND FOOD ALLERGY?

These terms are often used interchangeably but they have distinct and specific meanings:

* *Food hypersensitivity* is the umbrella term used to describe any reaction to food, encompassing both allergy and intolerance.
* *Food intolerance* describes a reaction to substances other than food proteins that do not involve the body's immune system. Many intolerances relate to a deficiency in specific enzymes which help digest certain foods. For example, lactose intolerance occurs when someone lacks the enzyme lactase and therefore can't digest the naturally occurring sugar in milk called lactose.
* *Food allergy* is the term reserved for reactions by the body's immune system to food proteins. These reactions can be either immediate or delayed.

IMMEDIATE IMMUNE MEDIATED FOOD ALLERGY

As the name suggests, these reactions happen quickly (within seconds or up to two hours after eating an allergen) and can, in some instances, be severe. They will result in one or more of the following symptoms:

* Skin (redness, eczema, hives, facial/ lip swelling)
* Gut (vomiting, diarrhoea)
* Respiratory tract (cough, wheeze, difficulty breathing, hoarseness, noisy breathing)
* Cardiovascular system (drop in blood pressure, profound drowsiness, lack of responsiveness or loss of consciousness)

- Anaphylaxis describes the most extreme form of an immediate allergic reaction where either difficulties breathing or a drop in blood pressure occur.

DELAYED IMMUNE MEDIATED FOOD ALLERGY

This is more difficult to diagnose as symptoms may occur one to three days after eating the relevant allergen. Some children are able to tolerate small amounts of the food protein but react to larger amounts, which can also complicate diagnosis. Typical symptoms can include one or more of the following:

- Eczema
- Vomiting
- Reflux
- Colic
- Abdominal pain
- Constipation
- Diarrhoea
- Blood or mucous in the stools
- Faltering growth

Additional symptoms such as lethargy, sleep disturbance and respiratory problems may relate to food allergies.

IS IT POSSIBLE TO HAVE A COMBINATION OF IMMEDIATE AND DELAYED REACTIONS?

Immediate and delayed food allergic reactions are quite distinct. However, they are not mutually exclusive. It is increasingly common for an individual to have delayed reactions to one or more food allergens as well as immediate reactions to others.

WHICH ARE THE MOST COMMON FOOD ALLERGIES?

Although any food protein has the potential to cause an allergic reaction, eight to ten foods account for 90 percent of all food allergic reactions. Eggs, cow's milk and nuts cause the most immediate reactions followed by wheat, sesame, kiwi, fish, shellfish and soya. Fewer foods cause delayed allergic reactions with cow's milk, soya, eggs and gluten causing the majority of problems.

IS IT UNUSUAL TO BE ALLERGIC TO SEVERAL DIFFERENT FOODS?

Up to two-thirds of children with allergies react to more than one food with some children being allergic to three or more of the common food allergens. Some food allergies are more commonly associated with others. Allergy to tree nuts and sesame occurs more frequently in children with peanut allergy and soya allergy is more prevalent in children with cow's milk allergy.

WILL MY CHILD OUTGROW HIS OR HER ALLERGY?

The good news is that about 80 per-cent of children who exhibit delayed reactions will grow out of their allergies by their third birthday. However, in a minority of cases, the symptoms can persist and should be thoroughly investigated.

With immediate reactions, it depends on the allergen in question. Tolerance is usually acquired over time with the majority of children outgrowing their allergies to milk, egg, wheat and soya by their 10th birthday. Allergy to nuts, sesame, fish and shellfish tend to be more persistent, with only a minority achieving tolerance in childhood. At least 80 percent of children with nut allergy remain allergic in adult life.

ARE THERE ANY TREATMENTS OR CURES FOR FOOD ALLERGY?

Treatments for food allergy are still experimental and not ready for use outside of established research programmes. The best strategy is food allergen avoidance and the provision of an emergency care plan supported with appropriate medications.

Allergy tests are helpful in the diagnosis of immediate food allergy. They also help determine when to introduce foods into your child's diet. Sometimes this will be done in hospital and sometimes it can be carefully managed at home following specific guidelines from your child's allergy specialist.

Avoiding multiple food groups poses challenges. A trained dietitian should always be involved to ensure that the prescribed diet really is free from the relevant allergens and is nutritionally adequate.

However, the real experts are the parents who live, shop, teach and cook for their allergic children. I am thrilled that two such parents have taken the time and effort to pass on some of their invaluable experience, gleaned through years of living with allergy.

They have gone the extra mile in providing recipes that will suit 90 percent of all allergic children, with recipes free from eight common allergens. I am sure this will become a valuable resource for many families who face the daunting daily prospect of coping with food allergy.

Food allergy is now relatively mainstream and no longer an uncommon condition. The good news about this is that it means you're not the only parent constantly reading labels and organising special food for parties and school trips.

We hope our advice will help to make your life easier in day-to-day situations. We really believe that food allergy needn't take over your life and you will quickly become used to checking labels and asking the right questions when eating away from home.

Your first few shopping trips may take a little longer than usual as you carefully read food labels and navigate the 'free-from' aisles, but you'll quickly get used to it. To help, we have given some information about each allergen and what typically to look out for when shopping for ingredients and food. However, our lists are by no means exhaustive and aim to give you a guide to the sorts of foods to check and be aware of from an allergen standpoint. Always seek guidance from your child's doctor or dietitian for more details on your child's specific needs.

We have also given you some tips for when you're out and about, based on our experience as parents of children with long-term multiple food allergies, that we hope you will find helpful.

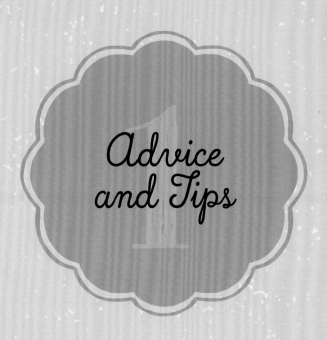

Advice
and Tips

FOOD LABELS

Once your child has been diagnosed with an allergy, it soon becomes second nature to check food labels when buying ingredients. Labelling in the UK and Europe is excellent. Food manufacturers must – by law – clearly highlight 14 major allergens (see box opposite) among the list of ingredients on packaging.

In December 2014 the rules on labelling in the EU changed and now all allergens need to be highlighted (in bold, underlined, or set in a larger font or in a different colour) in a list of ingredients. Do take care though, as we've noticed that on some labels the bold type (generally the preferred method of highlighting) doesn't always stand out clearly enough from the rest of the ingredients on the list so allergens can be missed.

FREE-FROM SUPERMARKET PRODUCTS

Products will often advertise the fact they are free from certain allergens on the front of the packet. They are rarely free from everything so you still need to check the label, but it can be useful to see at a glance if they exclude certain allergens.

TYPICAL LABEL HIGHLIGHTING ALLERGENS

Ingredients: **wheat** flour, fresh **butter** 29%, sugar, caramel 5% (glucose syrup, **butter**, sweetened concentrated **milk**, caramelised brown sugar and salt, emulsifier : lecithins [**soya**], natural flavouring), fresh **eggs**, sea salt, natural flavour, baking powder (sodium carbonates and diphosphates), skimmed **milk** powder.

May contain traces of sesame seeds and nuts.

THE EU's 14 MAJOR ALLERGENS

1 Milk

2 Eggs

3 Peanuts

4 Tree nuts (almonds, hazelnuts, walnuts, cashew, pecan, Brazil, pistachio, macadamia nuts)

5 Soya

6 Cereals containing gluten (wheat, oats, rye, barley, spelt and kamut)

7 Sesame

8 Fish

9 Molluscs

10 Crustaceans

11 Celery

12 Mustard

13 Sulphur dioxide and Sulphites

14 Lupin

'MAY CONTAIN' STATEMENTS

Food manufacturers often cover themselves if there is a big, or even a small, chance that food could have been contaminated with an allergen at any point in the production cycle. They use phrases such as:

* May contain traces of nuts
* Not suitable for milk/nut/egg allergy sufferers due to manufacturing methods
* Made in a factory that handles nuts

These statements are voluntary and are becoming more widespread. It is important to discuss with your child's doctor or dietitian if your child can eat products carrying these warnings. It's worth remembering that these warnings indicate a chance that the product is contaminated and even if your child has eaten a particular product before with no problem, there's no guarantee that the next one won't be contaminated.

Do remember to keep checking the labels of foods that you use repeatedly as ingredients and manufacturing processes change surprisingly frequently. Also be aware that labelling laws and terms that refer to allergens change so, as a parent, you need to keep abreast of the developments.

Take a look at our allergen sections where we list unusual foods in which you might not expect to find allergens. Scanning lists and unfamiliar vocabulary can be daunting at first. But you'll quickly get the hang of it. None of our lists of items to avoid or to be cautious of are exhaustive so you must always check every label carefully.

DAIRY

The term 'dairy' covers cow's milk and all of its many derivative products like butter, cheese and yoghurt. Goat, sheep and buffalo milks also need to be avoided as they contain similar allergenic proteins to cow's milk. Being allergic to dairy is different to being lactose intolerant and products that are suitable for those who are lactose intolerant must still be avoided by milk allergy sufferers as they still contain allergenic proteins.

LABELLING

Most commonly a label will list 'milk' or 'cow's milk' in bold but it is also possible for 'cheese', 'butter', 'cream' or 'yoghurt' to be highlighted on ingredient lists without reference to milk or cow's milk as these products are considered to be clearly derived from cow's milk and commonly used terms. Products such as mascarpone or ricotta could be shown on a label as mascarpone (**milk**) or could be shown as ricotta **cheese**.

If the vegan symbol appears on the product, this means it contains no animal products, including dairy, but do always check labels carefully for other allergens that your child may be allergic to.

WARNING:
FOODS TO AVOID
* Milk
* Cream
* Butter
* Cheese
* Yoghurt
* Ice cream
* Other animal milks (goat, sheep, buffalo)

CAUTION:
FOODS TO BE WARY OF
The following usually or sometimes contain dairy:
* Margarines, including sunflower and olive oil-based varieties
* Sausages, breaded or crumbed chicken, fish fingers
* Biscuits and cakes
* Chocolate, fudge, toffee
* Anything in batter or made from batter such as pancakes, Yorkshire puddings and tempura
* Soups and sauces such as béchamel and pesto
* Breakfast cereals
* Lactose-free foods and drinks (unless also dairy free)
* Popping candy
* Flavoured crisps

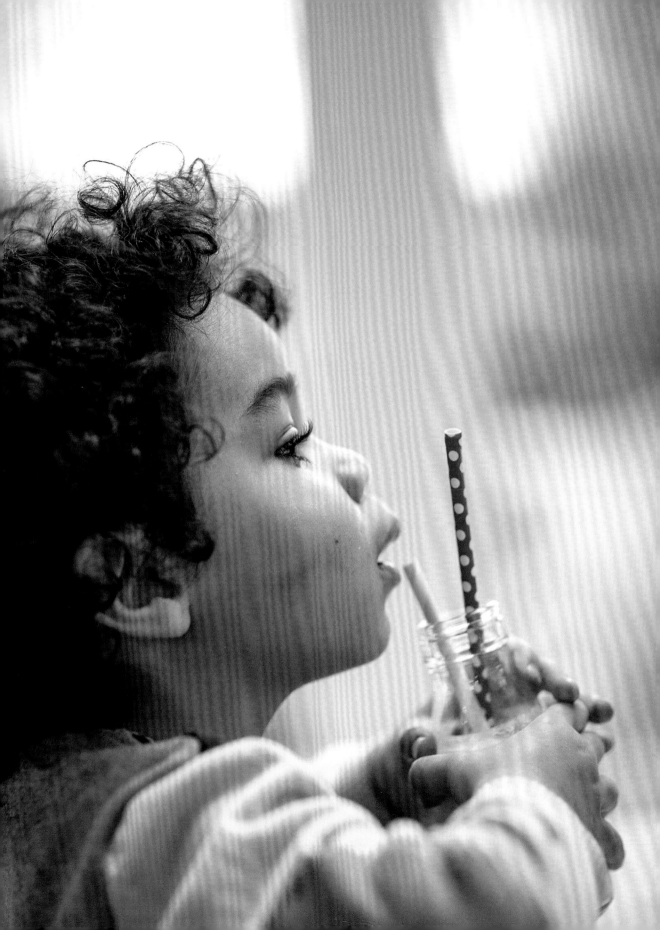

EGGS

Eggs are pretty handy things. Their physical properties – for example the fact that they solidify as they get hotter – mean that they are used as binding agents (to hold things together), emulsifiers (to stop water and oil in mayonnaise, for example, from separating), and aerators (to help trap air and lighten the texture in many baked goods).

People who are allergic to hen's eggs typically react to other eggs too, such as duck and quail eggs. Raw egg is the most allergenic form of egg, followed by cooked egg and lastly baked processed egg within foods such as cakes. There are many children who are allergic to eggs in any form. For this reason, all our recipes totally exclude eggs.

LABELLING
If a product that is being sold in the UK contains egg, it should be clearly labelled, as egg is classed as a major allergen. It's worth keeping a look-out for vegan symbols on food labels as these products shouldn't contain any animal products including egg but do check labels carefully for other allergens that your child may be allergic to.

WARNING:
FOODS TO AVOID
Eggs in all their forms:
* Poached
* Boiled
* Baked
* Fried
* Scrambled
* Omelette

CAUTION:
FOODS TO BE WARY OF
The following usually or sometimes contain egg:
* Cakes, pastry, biscuits and meringues
* Puddings, custards and mousses
* Royal icing and marzipan
* Sauces and condiments such as tartar, horseradish, béarnaise, hollandaise and mayonnaise
* Fresh egg pasta and noodles
* Ice cream and sorbets
* Sausages, burgers (veggie and meat), meatballs, fish fingers, anything that has a crumb coating
* Anything in batter or made from batter such as pancakes, Yorkshire puddings and tempura
* Stock cubes, gravy
* Marshmallows and chocolate confectionery
* Brioche, sweet buns, gluten-free bread, glazed rolls
* Meat substitutes (microprotein and soya-based varieties)

PEANUTS AND TREE NUTS

Peanuts aren't actually true nuts; they're part of the legume family and are therefore classified as groundnuts. Brazil nuts, hazelnuts, pistachio nuts, cashew nuts, pecan nuts, walnuts, macadamia nuts and almonds are all tree nuts.

LABELLING
Food containing nuts should be clearly highlighted on food labels. Labels will normally highlight the specific nut but sometimes simply 'nuts' will be highlighted in a product list. Many products use 'may contain traces of nuts' statements – see page 15 for more information.

WARNING:
FOODS TO AVOID
* Tree nuts (Brazil nuts, hazelnuts, pistachios, cashews, pecans, walnuts, macadamias and almonds)
* Peanuts
* Peanut butter
* Nut oils
* Satay
* Praline

CAUTION:
FOODS TO BE WARY OF
The following usually or sometimes contain nuts:
* Marzipan, nougat, chocolate bars, chocolate brownies
* Pre-packaged sauces, such as pesto and korma sauce
* Nut-based cakes and biscuits, such as Christmas cake
* Cereals and cereal bars
* Veggie burgers
* Ice cream
* Chocolate desserts
* Stir-fries and curries
* Middle Eastern sweets and desserts

SOYA

The soya bean belongs to the legume family, which includes peas, beans and peanuts. It is an extremely cheap source of both fat and protein – producing more of the latter per acre than any other food stuff. Soya is relatively easy to avoid in day-to-day cooking but is highly prevalent in processed foods – well over half of all manufactured foods contain soya in some form according to estimates.

LABELLING

Food labels normally state whether the product contains either soya or soya lecithin (E322).

Soya lecithin (E322) is often used as an emulsifier to stabilise foods that contain water and fats that do not normally mix. For example, it is used in most chocolate to stop the cocoa and cocoa butter from separating.

It is a fat which contains tiny traces of protein. It is rarely enough to cause a reaction, meaning most people with a soya allergy can tolerate soya lecithin. If so, there are many processed and manufactured foods that they will be able to eat but if not, labels will need to be checked very carefully. You need to establish with your child's doctor if your child can have foods containing soya lecithin.

WARNING:
FOODS TO AVOID

- Soya beans
- Soya milk, 'yoghurts' and puddings
- Tofu
- Soya-derived meat alternatives
- Miso
- Soya and tamari sauces
- Soya oil
- Edamame

CAUTION:
FOODS TO BE WARY OF

The following usually or sometimes contain soya protein or soya lecithin:

- Breakfast cereals
- Bread, cakes, pizza bases and biscuits
- Tinned soup
- Crackers, crisps
- Ready-made desserts, ice cream, chocolate
- Margarine
- Processed beef burgers, meat pies, minced beef, sausages and hotdogs
- Pancake and waffle mixes
- Pasta

GLUTEN

Gluten is present within grains such as wheat, barley, rye, spelt, kamut and in addition oats are often contaminated with gluten in their production process. Like eggs, gluten has an important role to play in baking – it helps cakes and dough to rise, giving them elasticity and structure. All the recipes in this book exclude all grains which contain gluten.

LABELLING AND GLUTEN-FREE PRODUCTS

Gluten-containing grains must be highlighted on food labels (normally as wheat, barley, etc. rather than highlighting gluten specifically). According to European labelling guidelines, for a product to be called 'Gluten-Free' it must contain no more than 20 parts of gluten per million. If a product states it is 'Very Low Gluten' it can contain no more than 100 parts of gluten per million.

Wheat and gluten-containing foods are key carbohydrates in many Western diets. You'll therefore have to be more inventive with carbohydrates your child can eat, like potatoes and rice. Have a look at our 'Potatoes and Rice' chapter for ideas.

WARNING:
FOODS TO AVOID
* Wheat, barley, rye, oats, spelt, kamut
* All baked goods containing wheat flour such as bread, cakes, biscuits, pastry, pizza bases etc.
* Porridge
* Pasta
* Couscous
* Semolina

CAUTION:
FOODS TO BE WARY OF
The following usually or sometimes contain gluten:
* Breakfast cereals
* Sausages, burgers, meatballs, fish fingers, coated chicken
* Anything in batter or made from batter such as pancakes, Yorkshire puddings and tempura
* White sauces like béchamel or cheese sauces with a roux (flour, butter, milk) base and other sauces
* Soya sauce
* Potato products like chips, crisps and roast potatoes can be lightly coated in flour to make them crispy
* Flavoured crisps
* Soups
* Gravy and stock cubes
* Baking powder
* Meat substitutes

SESAME

Sesame is used extensively in a variety of foods particularly as an oil, and it can often be found in Indian, Chinese, Japanese, Southeast Asian and Greek cuisines. It is commonly used to deep fry tempura, for pickling and in condiments as well as in hummus. The whole seeds are often used in baked goods.

LABELLING
As with all the 14 major allergens, sesame must be highlighted on food labels.

WARNING:
FOODS TO AVOID
* Sesame seeds
* Tahini paste
  (used in hummus)
* Sesame oil

CAUTION:
FOODS TO BE WARY OF
The following usually or sometimes contain sesame:
* Dips, especially Greek ones like aubergine dips and hummus
* Sausages, burgers, veggie burgers
* Margarines and spreads
* Chocolate bars and flapjacks
* Baked goods such as bread, buns, bagels, biscuits and breadsticks
* Salad dressings and chutneys
* Stir-fry sauces and curry sauces
* Garnishes on salads and vegetables
* Middle Eastern sweets and desserts

SHELLFISH

Shellfish can be divided into two main categories (see below). Even if your child is allergic to one type and not another you will need to be extremely careful to avoid cross contamination as different types of shellfish are often found close together on fish counters. Here are examples of commonly-found shellfish:

CRUSTACEANS
Prawns
Lobster
Crab
Crayfish
Shrimps
Langoustine
Scampi

MOLLUSCS
Are categorised into the following classes:

Gastropods
Periwinkles
Limpets
Abalone
Whelks
Snails (the edible type
found on land)

Bivalves
Mussels
Scallops
Clams (cockles)
Oysters
Cephalopods
Octopus
Squid
Cuttlefish

LABELLING
Food labels, according to European regulations, should clearly highlight whether a product contains a crustacean or a mollusc, for example: prawns (**crustacean**), mussels (**mollusc**).

If a product carries a Vegan symbol it should contain no animal products, including shellfish, but do check labels carefully for other allergens.

WARNING:
FOODS TO AVOID
* Crustaceans
* Molluscs
* Shellfish platters
* Fish soup (which uses shellfish as a base)
* Fish stock (which uses shellfish as a base)
* Paella

CAUTION:
FOODS TO BE WARY OF
The following usually or sometimes contain shellfish:
* Fish stock
* Fish soup (bouillabaise or marmite – fresh fish soup, not the spread)
* Sauces such as bisque, Oriental fish sauce, marinara sauce
* Pasta sauces (even tomato-based sauces can contain shellfish)
* Indian and Thai curry pastes
* Sushi (due to cross contamination)
* Dietary supplements, like fish oil, sometimes contain shellfish

OTHER ALLERGENS

Of the 14 major allergens that must be highlighted on ingredient lists according to EU regulations, the following four allergens *are* included in some of our recipes:

FISH

If your child is allergic to fish, you should be aware that we have included fish recipes in this book. We felt this was important as fish is such a good source of protein and oily fish, such as salmon and mackerel, provide Omega-3 fatty acids, which are important for brain and eye development.

Recipes containing fish are clearly labelled so that these dishes can be easily avoided if your child has a fish allergy. However, don't skip through them too quickly as we have suggested variations to replace the fish in many of these recipes. You can rest assured, that if you don't see the fish icon in the recipe heading, then no fish is contained in that particular recipe.

MUSTARD AND CELERY

We do include mustard and celery in a couple of recipes but they are optional so you can omit these ingredients if your child is allergic to them, without affecting the results.

SULPHITES

Sulphites or sulphur dioxide can sometimes be found in cured meat like ham and dried fruits. A couple of our recipes use cured meat such as Parma ham, dried apricots and raisins so check labels carefully when buying these foods or avoid these recipes if your child can't have sulphites.

LUPIN

This allergen is NOT included in any of our recipes. Lupin is not a common ingredient in the UK but is more prevalent in mainland Europe and is often used as a flour to replace gluten-containing grains (in gluten-free pasta for example). We do not include lupin or lupin flour in any of our recipes.

MYTH-BUSTING

✖ *Is it dairy?*
Cocoa butter is not derived from cow's milk and nor is cream of tartar, as their names may suggest.

✖ *Wheat or not wheat?*
Despite its name, buckwheat is not a grain – it is a fruit seed. Cornflour is not made from wheat and is gluten-free.

✖ *A nut or not a nut?*
Pine nuts and sweet chestnuts are technically classed as seeds. Similarly coconut is a fruit and water chestnut is an aquatic vegetable. Nutmeg is a spice.

ENJOYING LIFE
with Food Allergy

We each have a child with severe multiple food allergies and we have found that there's no need for them to miss out on everyday pleasures like eating out; and you do not have to worry constantly when they go off to nursery and school or when you're travelling. By taking a few precautions there's really no need to panic about food allergy and once you get into the swing of things, it's very straightforward.

EATING OUT

Of course we do lots of cooking at home but we also love eating out with our children and there's no reason why children with food allergies shouldn't enjoy this experience too. Here are a few tips based on our personal experience.

WHERE CAN YOU EAT?

Some restaurants are better suited than others at catering for people with food allergies: those with simpler menus where the food is carefully prepared on the premises are usually good choices. It is worth bearing in mind that depending on your child's set of allergies some cuisines may not be ideal and as such we have given recipes from cuisines from all around the world that you can prepare easily and eat safely at home.

PHONE AHEAD

It is a good idea to warn the restaurant that you're coming as they're often happy to accommodate dietary needs and will sometimes make you something special if they're given some notice. It is a requirement of the labelling regulations that restaurants and delis now highlight allergens either via a menu, chalkboard or verbally via a waiter or waitress.

ASK THE RIGHT QUESTIONS

Ensure you ask the right questions when you're eating out and get clear answers. We both have experience of being told something is free from dairy or gluten or egg or sesame. But when we ask more specific questions such as 'Is there any butter or cream used in the sauce?'; 'Has butter been added to the vegetables?'; 'Is egg used to bind the burger or glaze the bun?'; 'Are there breadcrumbs in the sausages?'; or 'What type of cooking oil has been used?' the reality can turn out to be different. In our individual allergen sections we've listed foods where you might not expect to find allergens – we hope this will help you ask the right questions.

ORDER SOMETHING SIMPLE

As a general rule it is worth ordering things with as few ingredients as possible. For example grilled chicken is a safer option than complicated dishes – especially those with sauces – which are more likely to contain allergens that aren't immediately obvious.

DOUBLE CHECK INGREDIENTS

Remember to ask about ingredients every time you visit a restaurant even if you eat there regularly as kitchens often change the ingredients and suppliers they use.

CLEAN SURFACES

Without overstating or being too cautious, it's worth wiping down high chairs and table tops as there is often residue left on surfaces even if they look quite clean. Especially in the case of severe allergies – it really is better to be safe than sorry. We once had to leave a restaurant because Isabelle's arms and face were covered in hives and if your child is at risk of an anaphylactic reaction, it's particularly important to take precautions.

DAYS OUT

It's always best to take something for your child to eat if you're out for the day. We find that some venues make fantastic provision for children with allergies. But other places – such as many theme parks and museums – find it more difficult to be accommodating. It's often hard to know whether a venue will be able to cater for your child before you get there, and by then, of course, it's too late. We've found that in the vast majority of cases, if a venue isn't easily able to make something for your child, they are more than happy for your child to eat something you've brought with you. The rest of you are paying after all!

We generally keep some snacks on us at all times. That way, if we're ever delayed, we've always got something to give the children. This is invaluable when your children are small and prone to tantrums when they're hungry. A pot of Fruit Salad (see page

219), some Banana Bread (see page 208), or Jam Tarts (see page 213) are all good ideas.

TRAVELLING

Travelling with young children can be a bit of a nightmare regardless of whether or not they have food allergies. If your children have food allergies it's wise to be just that bit more organised about the food you bring for them. We suggest always bringing more than you need.

Travelling by car tends to be relatively easy because you can pack what you need and take plenty of snacks and fruit in case of unexpected delays. You don't want to rely on service station food; it's very difficult to find sandwiches without butter and near impossible to find gluten-free bread.

Service stations often have microwaves in the restaurant seating areas. We tend to take frozen portions of things like risotto or casseroles in a cool bag for an easy but substantial meal on a long journey. Good recipes include our No-Fuss Butternut Squash Risotto (see page 45), Comforting Chicken Casserole (see page 51), Creamy Courgette Risotto (see page 40) and our Lentil and Vegetable Stew (see page 98).

Travelling on a plane can be a little more problematic, particularly as there are strict rules about carrying liquids and gels on board. It is always useful to carry a doctor's letter outlining the child's allergy as we've found airport security officials tend to be more understanding if you can produce one.

Some airlines do provide free-from meals. Personally, we feel that the last place you want your children to have an allergic reaction is 30,000 feet up in the air and hours from the nearest hospital. So now's not the time to be taking a chance on an untried source.

Cold food that you can put in one tub is a good option when you're travelling by plane. You can try our Three Bean Salad (see page 142), Rice Salad (see page 143), Sushi (see page 198), Gluten-Free Pasta Salad (see page 145) or Green Vegetable and Quinoa Salad (see page 150) as they're all substantial, filling meals but don't need heating up and are easy to eat with a fork or spoon straight from the tub.

As with restaurants, it's worth wiping down tray tables and asking airline staff to vacuum any crumbs or nuts around your seats and dissuade your child from putting their hands down the sides of seats where debris often collects.

AVOIDING ALLERGEN CROSS CONTAMINATION AT HOME

You can easily avoid cross contamination of allergens at home by taking some simple precautions:

* Use separate spoons and knives for jams and spreads. Alternatively, ensure your allergic child has their own jars or tubs of spreads that no one else touches.
* Try and keep allergen-free items like special milk, spreads and jams on a separate shelf away from allergens like milk and butter.
* For those who are seriously allergic to gluten-containing grains, it might be worth considering getting a separate toaster.
* Be scrupulous with cloths and ensure that you don't use one to wipe up an allergen that might be used for your allergic child before it has been carefully rinsed with soap and hot water. We tend to use different coloured cloths.
* It can be a little tricky when you have one child who is allergic and another who isn't. This is the case for both of us. We generally give Casper and his sister Camille and Isabelle and her sister Zara the same free-from main meals but both of us will give things like bread, cheese and yoghurts to our younger, non-allergic, children and these can be messy – especially when the children are little. We tend to get the children to sit at opposite sides of the table and make sure that all children wash their hands as soon as they leave the table and before they touch anything else.

LEAVING YOUR CHILDREN IN THE CARE OF OTHERS

School, Nursery, Summer Camps, Clubs and Parties

At the best of times it's hard to hand responsibility for your child to someone else. And it can be even more worrying if your child has a serious food allergy. But, if you're prepared and have a good relationship with your child's school, nursery or club, there's no reason why everything shouldn't go smoothly. Ask lots of questions as it's important you feel comfortable and confident that others will handle your child's allergy appropriately. Below are a few questions you may like to ask, particularly when your child is starting school or if they have been invited to a party.

DOES THE SCHOOL HAVE A PROTOCOL OR STRATEGY FOR DEALING WITH FOOD ALLERGY?

Most schools and nurseries are used to dealing with allergies and children with restricted diets. Many have clearly laid out protocols and the majority of schools we've spoken to have specific policies on nuts.

WHERE WILL MEDICATION BE KEPT? WHO WILL ADMINISTER IT?

Bring a doctor's treatment plan to school outlining how and in what circumstances different medication should be used and when an ambulance should be called. Agree on a plan for your child that both you and your child's teachers feel comfortable with.

ARE ALL MEMBERS OF STAFF TRAINED TO USE AN ADRENALINE AUTO-INJECTOR?

It's very important to ensure that class teachers and staff looking after your child have a good grasp of which foods to avoid and also feel confident to administer medication, including adrenaline auto-injectors, should that ever be necessary.

CAN YOU DISCUSS YOUR CHILD'S DIETARY REQUIREMENTS WITH THE CATERING STAFF AND WILL THEY NEED A PACKED LUNCH?

Many schools, like ours, are happy for you to discuss menus directly with catering staff and will be happy to show you preparation areas so you can be confident that there won't be cross contamination. If you prefer to or need to make packed lunches for your child every day, do look at our packed lunches section (see page 240). This will give you some ideas for ensuring your child gets a varied menu and that you don't have to rack your brains every morning to think of what to put in their lunchbox.

WHAT HAPPENS ON SCHOOL TRIPS OR WHEN PLAYING SPORTS MATCHES AWAY FROM SCHOOL?

Once your child is a bit older and goes to clubs, summer camps, sports matches and other events, you'll need to make sure the staff are aware of the food allergy especially if there's going to be food prepared by another school or provider. In this situation we always recommend sending your child with a packed tea/snack. Have a look at our packed lunches section for some ideas (see page 240).

FIND OUT WHAT COOKING ACTIVITIES AND OTHER CHILDREN'S BIRTHDAYS ARE PLANNED FOR THE TERM

It will make a big difference if you offer to help your school by providing special recipes or ingredients when the class is baking or cooking. We often email classmates' parents to find out when they are planning to bring in cakes for birthdays so we can bring in something suitable for our children. We always have a batch of cupcakes in the freezer that we can defrost as and when we need them (see page 210). The children's class teachers also have a supply of dairy-free chocolate buttons just in case we forget.

WHAT ABOUT BAKE SALES?

Bake sales are clearly a challenge. We generally make something special for our own children to buy – not the best business model, but it means that there's something there for other allergy sufferers too. Our Chocolate Refrigerator Cake (see page 225), Chocolate Crispie Cakes (see page 226) and Chocolate Cake (see page 210) are popular choices with all the children – allergic or not.

WHAT WILL THEY EAT AT PARTIES?

Don't worry about bothering the parent of the child whose party it is as they probably have a lot to organise and think about. Our children's friends and their parents are very understanding of our children's allergies but we are conscious that we don't want to make life difficult for them. We generally bring food for our children to eat at parties, especially if it is being held at friends' houses. As for venues, it can sometimes be useful to phone ahead and ask about the menu or see if they can prepare something special for you. Remember to check any party bags for cake, chocolate or anything else so that you can fish them out before your child starts delving inside.

WHAT ABOUT THEIR MEDICATION AT PARTIES?

When you drop children off at parties rather than stay with them, it's important to ensure their medication is left at the party venue and someone at the party knows what to do in case of an allergic reaction. We normally just talk to the parents well in advance of the party to explain how to use an adrenaline auto-injector and ensure they are happy to administer it in the unlikely event it is needed. We both also always ensure we're easily contactable and nearby in case of emergency.

EDUCATION ABOUT ALLERGY

Making your child aware of his or her allergies is very important and can be done from a very young age. Key points we feel are important to get across include:

* Always tell adults about your allergies.
* Don't automatically trust that an adult will understand allergies.
* Always ask adults to check labels (if your child can't yet read) or check labels.
* Alert an adult if you think you have eaten something containing an allergen.
* Never share food.
* Remember to wash hands before eating.
* Alert an adult if you think you are having an allergic reaction.

It is useful to see how your child reacts when he or she is offered a food they shouldn't have. Consider not intervening before your child has had a chance to refuse the food themselves or to ask what's in it. From a young age Isabelle and Casper would refuse food and explain: 'I am allergic'. They generally get lots of sympathetic attention when they do this (especially when they explain that they can't have cake or ice cream), so it has actually become a positive experience. In fact, we suspect they're starting to milk it a little! We both find that our children repeat the phrases they've heard us use and we tend to be consistent in how we ask about ingredients and how we explain our children's allergies.

Rather than just getting your child to say that they are allergic to dairy or gluten, make sure they understand what that means and which products contain the ingredients to which they are allergic. It's surprising how many adults forget there is usually butter in biscuits or sesame in hummus. Equally, it's surprising how quickly even quite small children can learn what they can and can't eat. It's also important that your child understands the severity of his or her allergy. We have experienced well-meaning adults telling our allergic children that they are also 'allergic' to dairy only to go on to eat a whole bowl of ice cream in front of them. Our children understand that some people have intolerances, meaning they mostly avoid a food but can eat it sometimes. They both understand that this is not the case for them and that they must never eat the foods they are allergic to as they would be extremely unwell if they did.

Also ensure that non-allergic siblings understand food allergy so that they are careful if they are eating allergens near their allergic brothers or sisters.

As children get older it's important that they start to take responsibility for looking after their own medication and ensuring they always have it with them.

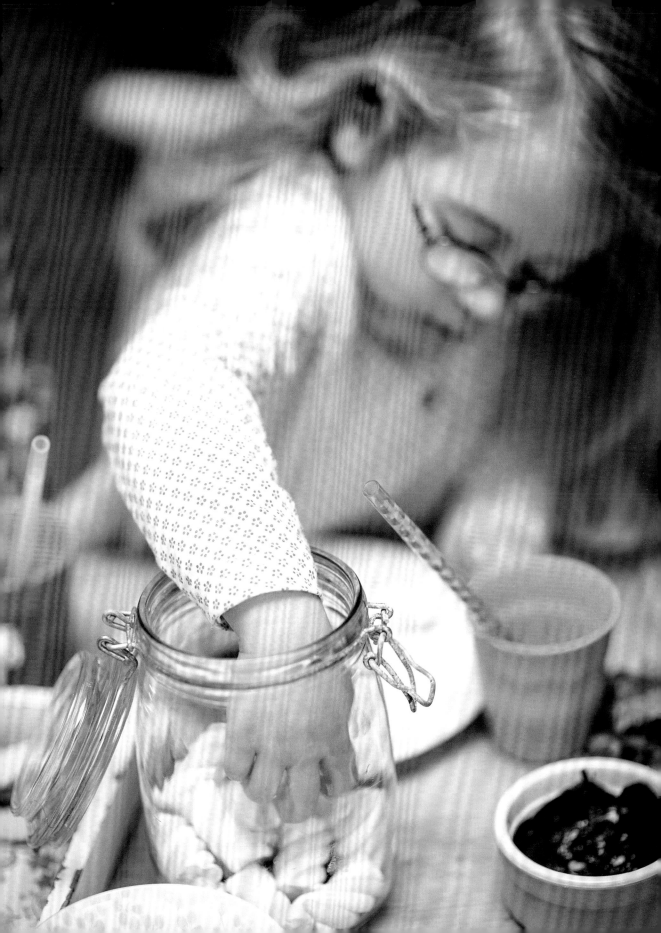

INFORMATION IS KEY

Don't assume people are aware of the seriousness of food allergy or your child's particular circumstances and don't expect teachers, staff and friends to think of everything. Try to make sure your child has a good grasp of which foods they're allergic to and encourage them to take responsibility for avoiding foods they can't eat. Isabelle and Casper understand that they can't always join in with everything. We are generally able to make up for this at home and, on the whole, we don't feel they miss out.

OUR FOOD PHILOSOPHY

✳ Food allergies should do nothing to prevent your child's full enjoyment of life.
✳ Anyone should be able to make our allergy-safe, straightforward, nutritious but delicious recipes.
✳ We firmly believe in making healthy food appealing to children and still tasty for parents who like to eat with their kids.
✳ We want to make it quick and easy for everyone with a child with an allergy to provide them with a healthy, balanced, varied and interesting diet.
✳ We advocate simple, easy-to-obtain, good quality (organic and sustainable where possible) ingredients.
✳ Cooking with kids and having fun with food can help to reduce anxiety about allergen avoidance.

USING THIS BOOK

We have tried to make our recipes straightforward from a cooking perspective and also from a food allergy point of view.

KEY TO THE RECIPES

! We have used this symbol throughout the book as a little reminder to check ingredient labels on manufactured or processed products that are used in some of our recipes. Most of the time these products will be free from allergens but certain brands sometimes do add them (from our excluded list of eight common allergens) so it's important to check labels to find a brand that's suitable. For example some brands of stock cube contain egg and/or celery. Some brands of chocolate that are dairy-free, contain soya lecithin or may contain traces of nuts so ! in an ingredient list reminds you to check the label.

Many recipes make suggestions for additional or substitute ingredients.

If you are not allergic
Additional ingredients
suggested here

We always highlight recipes that contain fish

VARIATION

Some recipes, particularly those with fish, offer alternatives such as chicken, lamb or vegetarian options.

A NOTE ON SALT

Children should eat a lot less salt than adults. Most people will eat a lot of salt in processed foods. Typically high salt levels are found in foods such as stock cubes, ham, smoked fish, ready meals, ketchups, cheese, bread products and some breakfast cereals to name a few.

Salt is only mentioned in a couple of our recipes where we feel it is an important ingredient, but it is entirely optional. A lot of our recipes have fresh herbs and other lovely flavours that mean you will not need to add salt to improve the taste – they are delicious already.

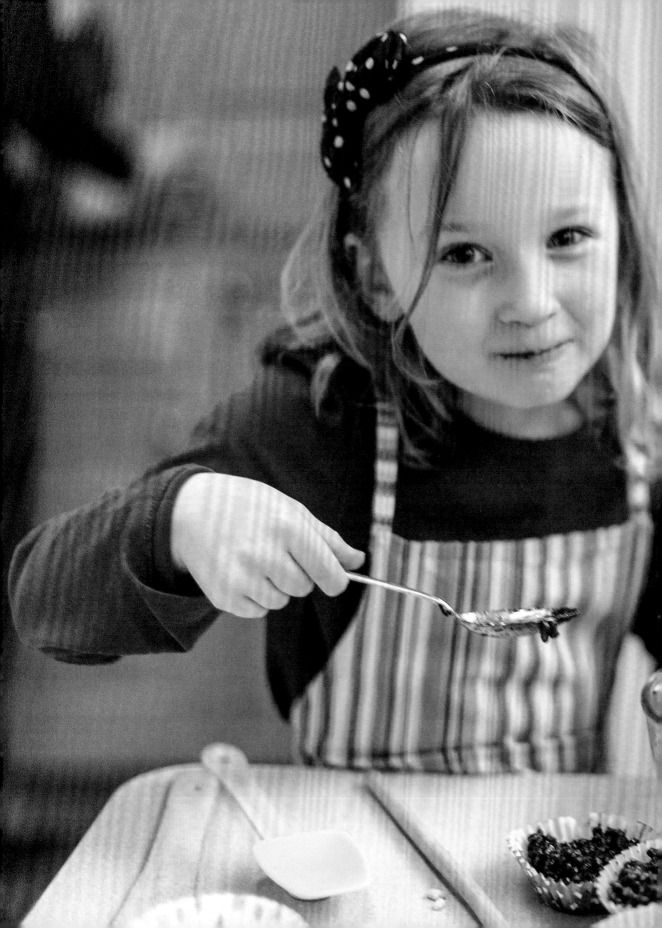

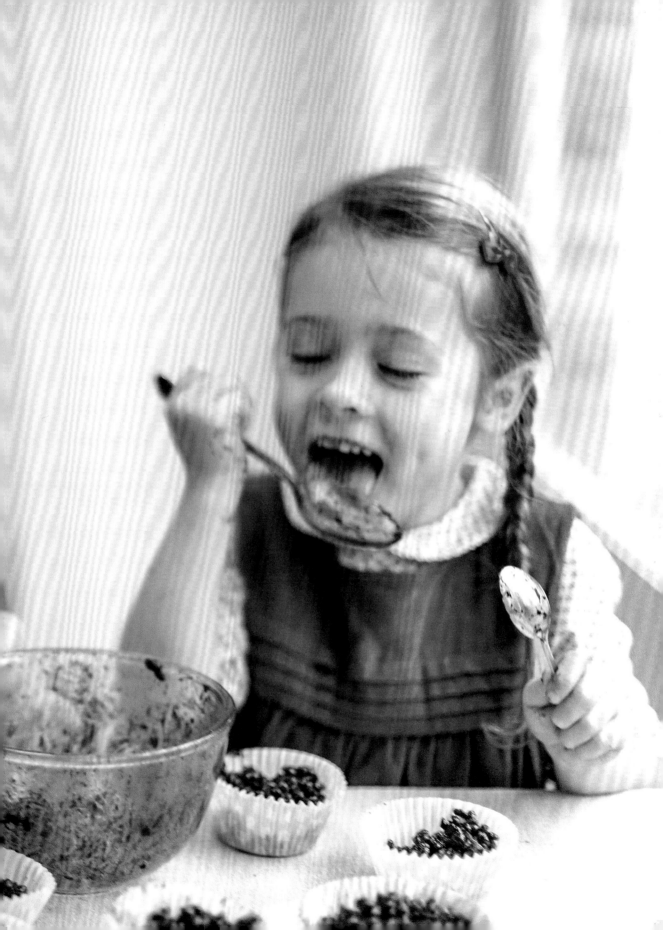

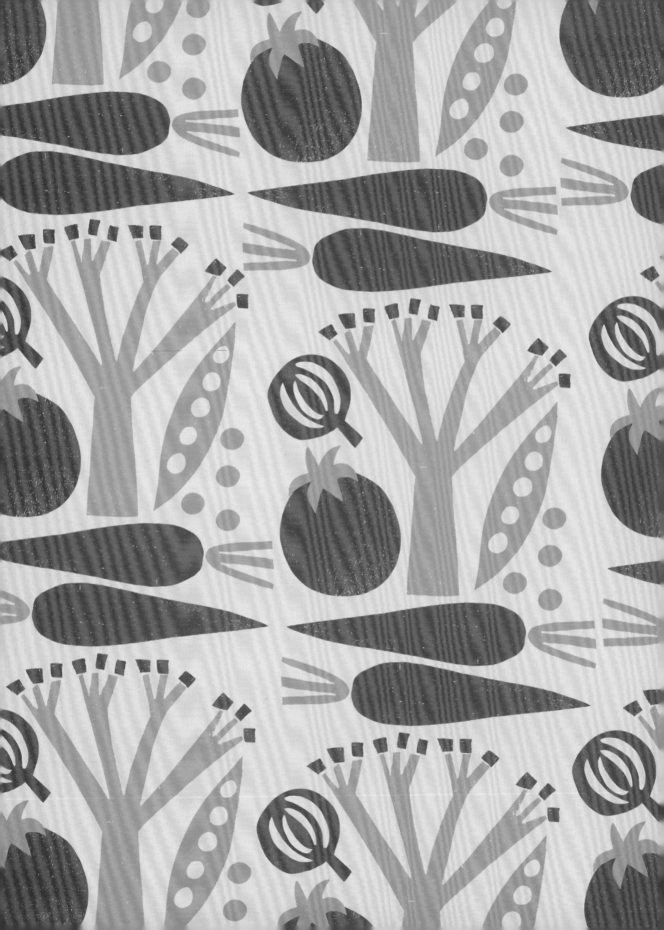

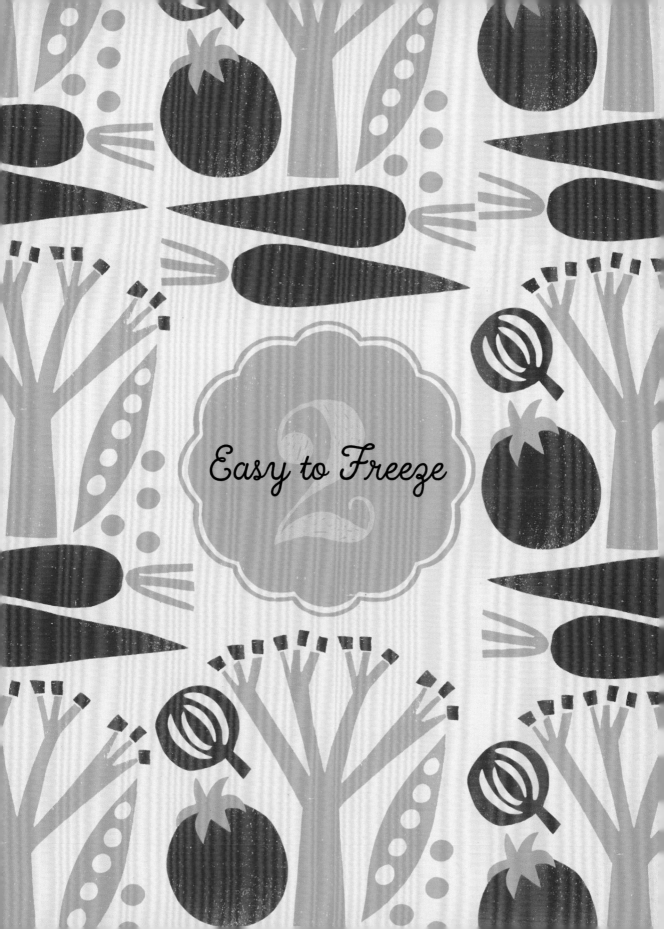

Easy to Freeze

2

We got into the habit of making big batches of food for the freezer when our children were babies and we were making lots of baby purée. It's a habit that stuck and we still regularly make large quantities of food to freeze. It can be a real timesaver to have lots of pre-made food in the freezer so that you don't have to cook every day. Having options in the freezer means it's easy to whip something out at the last minute when you're in a rush or need to cater for unexpected guests. It's great when you're too busy to cook but you still know you can produce home-cooked, allergy-safe meals in an instant.

This is a selection of recipes that you can make in advance, freeze in portion sizes to suit you and your family and then just defrost in the microwave and heat up when you want a quick meal. We tend to freeze in portions to feed two children as we each have two children and smaller portions are quick to defrost. Find a system to suit you and your family and make the most out of your freezer.

These recipes are equally good eaten the same day. We often make more than we need for one meal and then freeze any that is left over.

FREEZING TIPS

We often buy freezer bags with zip locks. This allows you to fill the bag, flatten it out and pop it into the freezer, maximising space. It can also be very handy to freeze food portions in little tubs and then they can be washed and re-used.

We find it useful to have a range of plastic tubs of all shapes and sizes anyway, for storing, transporting and freezing food in. By using tubs you know the food is contained and sealed and not going to come into contact with anything else. If you use tubs to store portions of food, ensure the food is totally cooled before sealing the lid on.

When you're ready to eat the frozen food, defrost it thoroughly. You can defrost portions of food overnight in a fridge or use a defrost setting on the microwave. Any food that has been frozen can only be safely reheated once and not multiple times and it is essential to check the food is piping hot throughout before serving.

GUIDELINES FOR FREEZING

The basic rule is to allow food to cool down to room temperature quickly before freezing.

* Cool any food to room temperature as quickly as you can and then put it in the freezer.
* Don't leave food in the pan to cool down, use a shallow dish and spread it out or put it into the smaller containers you plan to freeze it in.
* Do not put hot or warm food in the freezer.

Once in the freezer, food should usually be eaten within one to three months.

SERVES A FAMILY OF

4

generously

PREP: 5 MINUTES
COOK: 30 MINUTES

Our kids love risotto. It is a filling and comforting meal that is easy to make and requires just one pan. This risotto is great for those with dairy allergy as it tastes and looks really creamy. It is the grated courgette that melts away in the cooking process that creates the creamy texture.

Creamy COURGETTE RISOTTO

2 tablespoons olive oil,
   plus extra to drizzle
2 unsmoked bacon
   rashers, chopped
½ small onion,
   finely chopped
1 garlic clove, crushed
250g risotto rice
   (Carnaroli or Vialone
   Nano are best as they
   give a creamy result)
1 litre Vegetable Stock
   (see page 248) or
   1 low-salt vegetable
   stock cube **!** dissolved
   in 1 litre boiling water
1 large courgette, grated
16 cherry tomatoes,
   halved
Balsamic vinegar,
   to drizzle
Freshly ground black
   pepper

1 Heat the oil in a heavy-based pan. Add the bacon and fry over a medium heat for 5 minutes until lightly browned. Add the onion and allow it to soften for a minute, then add the garlic and rice. Give it a stir to make sure the rice does not stick to the bottom of the pan.

2 When the rice starts to glisten, add a ladleful of stock, then add the courgette and stir well until all the stock has been absorbed by the rice.

3 Add another ladleful of stock and stir until the rice has absorbed it, then add another. Keep doing this at intervals, stirring for about 15–18 minutes until the rice is tender but still firm to bite.

4 If you use all your stock and feel more liquid is needed to finish cooking the rice, just use a little extra water.

5 Remove from the heat, stir in the cherry tomatoes, season to taste and let the risotto rest in the pan for a few minutes. Spoon into bowls and drizzle with a little olive oil and balsamic vinegar.

> *If you are not allergic*
> Add a handful of grated
> Parmesan cheese at
> the end of cooking.

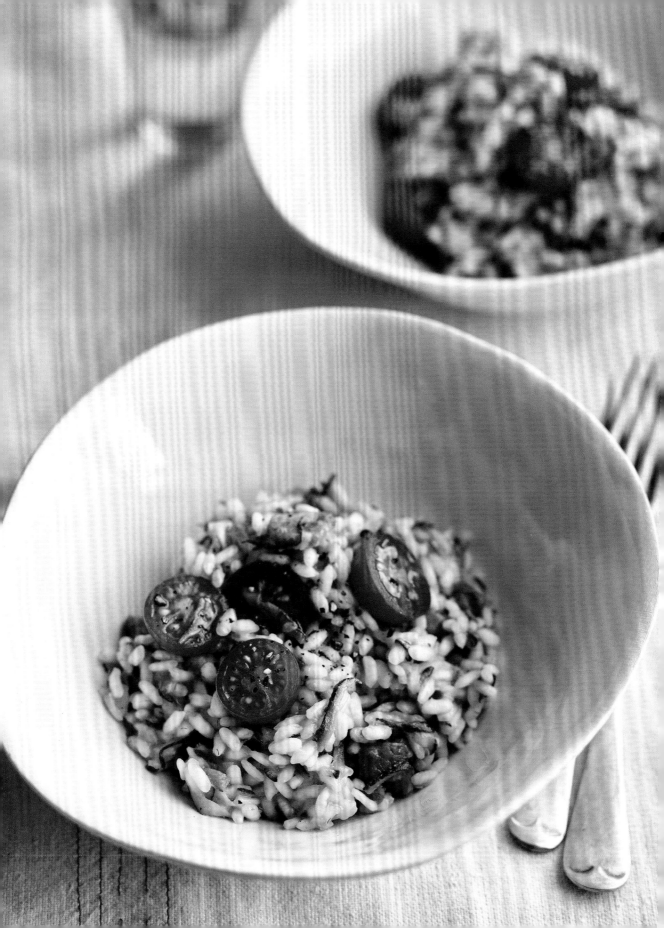

PREP: 5 MINUTES
COOK: 25 MINUTES

This tomato-based sauce is great for fussy eaters as it has lots of fruit and vegetables concealed within it, contributing to the five different fruit and vegetables we should all eat every day. The fruit in the sauce gives it a little sweetness that appeals to kids so it is usually a huge hit with those children who aren't keen on eating their vegetables. The sauce is lovely with gluten-free pasta and also works well as a sauce to accompany a piece of plain grilled meat and is the perfect accompaniment to our Pork Meatballs (see page 90).

Five-a-Day PASTA SAUCE

1 tablespoon olive oil
1 small onion, chopped
1 garlic clove, crushed
400g tin chopped
    tomatoes
2 teaspoons tomato purée
300ml water
2 good handfuls curly
    kale (about 120g)
4 baby sweetcorn
6 dried apricots
1 carrot, peeled and
    roughly chopped
15 seedless grapes
Freshly ground
    black pepper

1 Heat the oil in a saucepan over a medium heat. Add the onion and cook for about 2–3 minutes until softened. Add the garlic and give it a good stir.

2 Add all the remaining ingredients to the pan, stir together and simmer gently for 20 minutes.

3 Remove from the heat and leave the sauce to cool.

4 Blend the sauce using a liquidiser or hand-held blender. We like to stop before it is totally smooth so you can still see flecks of the different vegetables. Adjust the consistency of the sauce to personal taste, adding a little water if needed.

Optional Extras
You can play around with the ingredients and add whatever vegetables you happen to have to hand. Peas, butternut squash, broccoli and red peppers all work well.

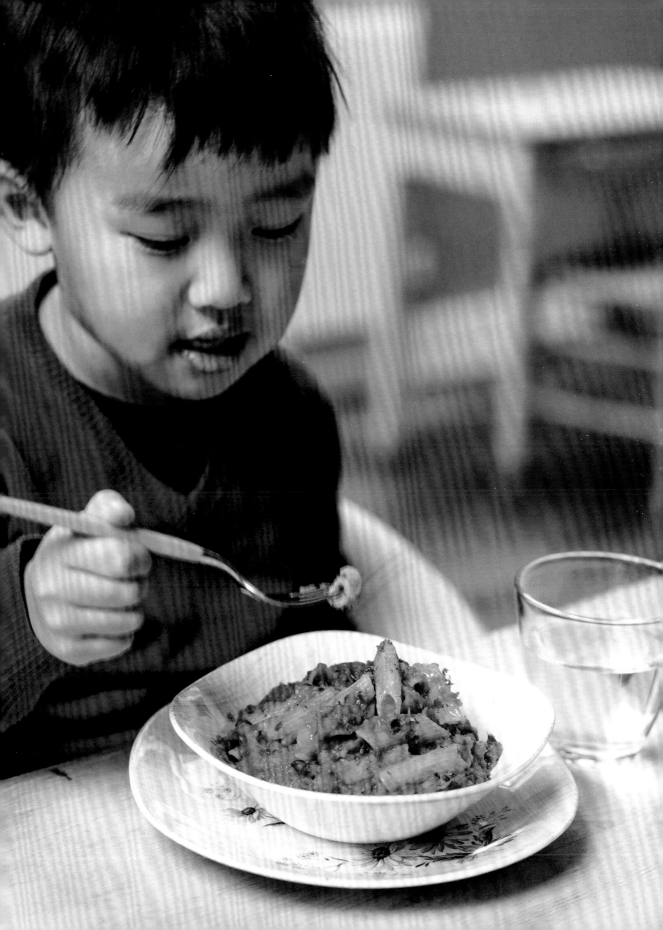

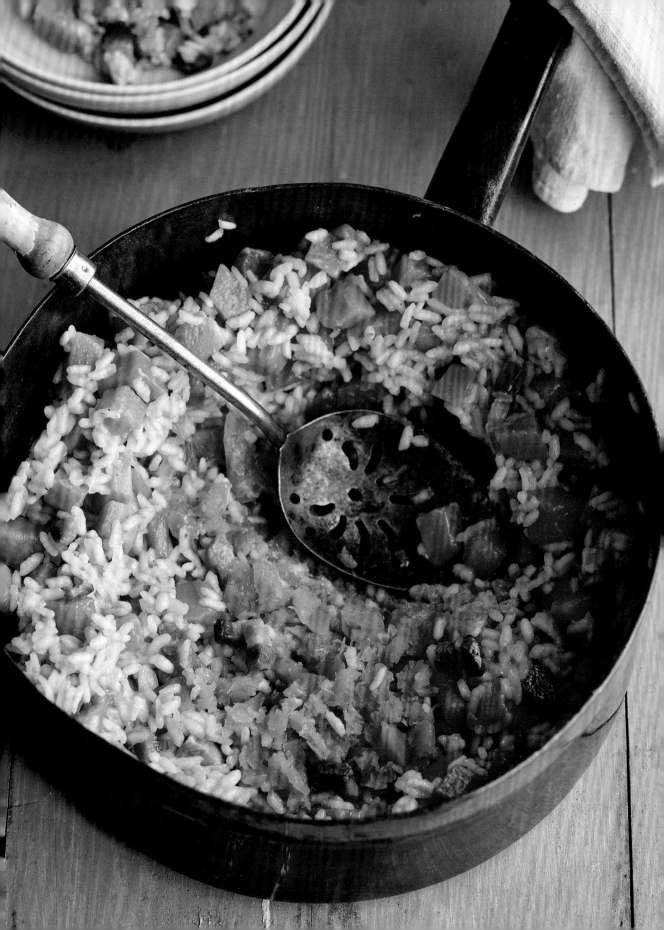

SERVES A FAMILY OF 4 *generously*

PREP: 5 MINUTES
COOK: 30 MINUTES

Most risottos require you to stand at the hob and stir the rice as it cooks but this risotto doesn't need constant attention, allowing you to get on with other things. You can let it simmer away with just the occasional stir. Freeze in portions to suit your family. Once defrosted, reheat adding just a little water to bring it back to the right consistency. This is Zara's favourite recipe and she would eat it every day if she could.

No-Fuss
BUTTERNUT SQUASH RISOTTO

2 tablespoons olive oil, plus extra to drizzle
2 unsmoked bacon rashers, chopped
½ small onion, finely chopped
1 garlic clove, crushed
250g risotto rice (Carnaroli is best)
1 litre Vegetable Stock (see page 248) or 1 low-salt vegetable stock cube ❗ dissolved in 1 litre boiling water
1 butternut squash, peeled, deseeded and cut into cubes
Balsamic vinegar, to drizzle
Freshly ground black pepper

1 Heat the oil in a heavy-based pan over a medium-high heat. Add the bacon and cook for about 5 minutes until lightly browned. Add the onion and allow it to soften for a minute or two.

2 Stir in the garlic and rice. Keep stirring so nothing sticks to the bottom of your pan and when the rice starts to glisten add all of the stock and the butternut squash. Bring to a gentle simmer.

3 Stir occasionally and cook for about 15–18 minutes until the rice is tender but still has a little bite to it. If you use up all your stock and feel some extra liquid is needed to finish cooking the rice, just add a little water.

4 Remove from the heat and break up the butternut squash into the risotto using a fork, or very gently press down using a potato masher. Season to taste and let the risotto rest in the pan for a few minutes.

5 Spoon into bowls and drizzle with a little olive oil and balsamic vinegar.

> *If you are not allergic*
> Stir in a generous handful of grated Cheddar cheese at the end of cooking.

Although this doesn't have a dairy-based white sauce like a traditional fish pie, it retains many of the same comforting qualities and is a lot easier to make. When buying fish, check to see it comes from a sustainable source. Pollock, coley, haddock, salmon and trout all work well either on their own or you can use a combination.

Easy Peasy FISH PIE

1 teaspoon olive oil

¼ small onion, finely chopped

750g floury potato (such as Maris Piper), peeled and roughly chopped into small chunks

½ courgette, chopped into small chunks

500g any firm white fish of your choice, bones and skin removed and cut into chunks

100g frozen peas

Splash of white wine vinegar

Small handful fresh parsley, finely chopped

2 tomatoes, chopped into chunks

Juice of ½ lemon

Freshly ground black pepper

1 Heat the oil in a saucepan over a medium heat. Add the onion and cook for about 3 minutes until softened.

2 Add the potato and courgette, cover with water and cook for a further 5–10 minutes until the potato feels soft.

3 Drain using a sieve and then mash lightly using a potato masher. It is good to keep a few lumps so the mash isn't too smooth, giving the pie a nice texture.

4 Place the fish in a separate pan and just cover with water. Add a splash of white wine vinegar and simmer very gently over a low heat for 3–5 minutes until the fish is cooked. Add the frozen peas to the cooking fish for the last 30 seconds or so.

5 Drain the peas and fish over a bowl just so you can keep a few tablespoons of the cooking liquid.

6 Mix the peas, fish and 2 tablespoons of the cooking liquor into the mashed potato. Add the parsley, chopped tomatoes and lemon juice; mix through and season to taste with black pepper.

7 Spoon the mixture into a large ovenproof dish or individual dishes. Pop under a preheated hot grill for a few moments until the top takes on a little colour.

If you are not allergic
Add a little grated cheese to the mixture and on top before grilling.

Optional Extras
Chopped capers are a great addition for extra flavour and can be added at the same time as the parsley.

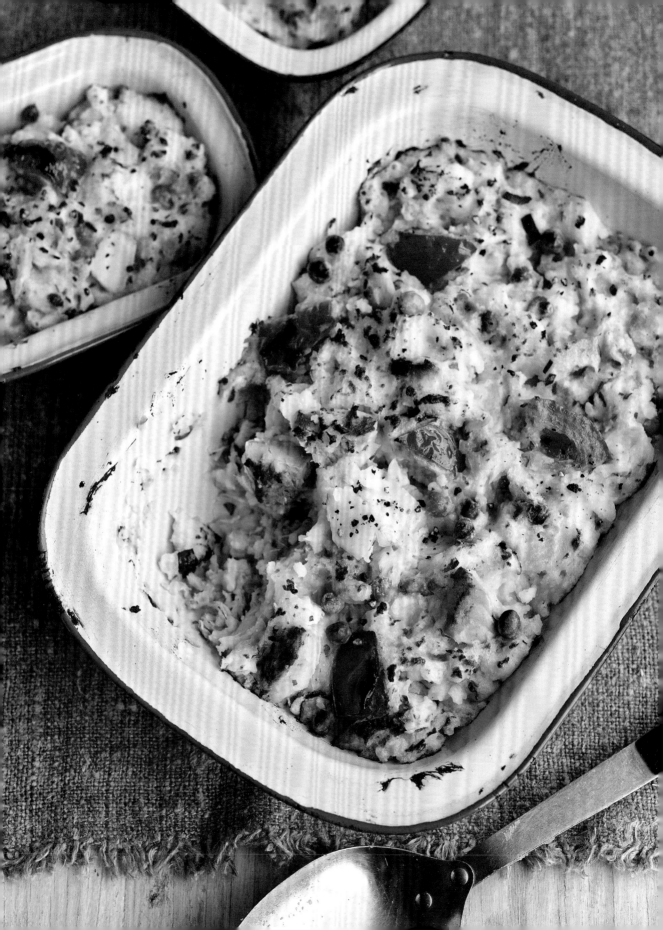

SERVES A FAMILY OF 4

PREP: 5 MINUTES
COOK: 15 MINUTES

This curry is not spicy but lovely and creamy and full of Thai flavours and aromas. You'll need to have some of our Homemade Southeast Asian Blend (see page 251) to hand to add the essential herbs and spices, but this only takes a few minutes to whip up and you can freeze it in batches so you've always got some whenever you need it. This curry is a real favourite with all the children and a popular mid-week supper. It is great simply served with some boiled rice and lime wedges.

Mild Thai Coconut CHICKEN CURRY

Drizzle of olive oil

3 tablespoons Homemade Southeast Asian Blend (see page 251)

2 x 400g tins coconut milk

3 skinless chicken breasts, sliced into pieces

16 baby sweetcorn, cut into rounds

1 courgette, quartered lengthways and then sliced

Small broccoli head, broken into small bite-size pieces

2 pak choi bulbs, sliced lengthways

2 large handfuls frozen peas

Small handful fresh coriander, finely chopped

1 Heat a little oil in a frying pan or saucepan. Add the Southeast Asian Blend and cook over a medium heat for about 3 minutes until the shallot in the mix has softened.

2 Add the coconut milk and bring to a gentle simmer.

3 Add the chicken, sweetcorn, courgette, broccoli and pak choi, then simmer for about 5 minutes or until the chicken is just cooked.

4 Add the frozen peas and cook for 30 seconds or so.

5 Garnish with the coriander.

....

Optional Extras
If your child needs feeding up, use a tin or carton of coconut cream as well as the coconut milk.

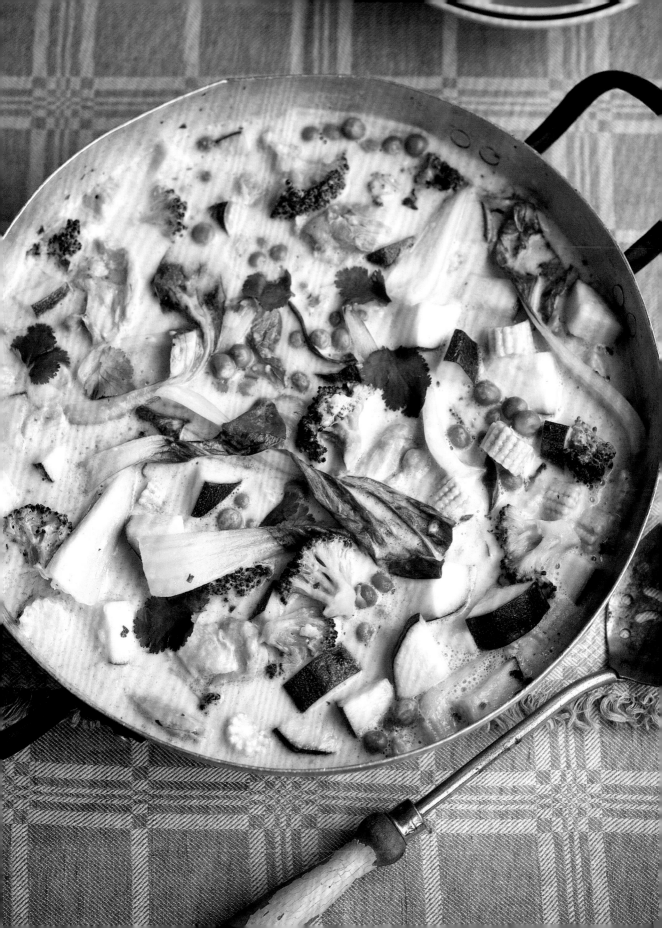

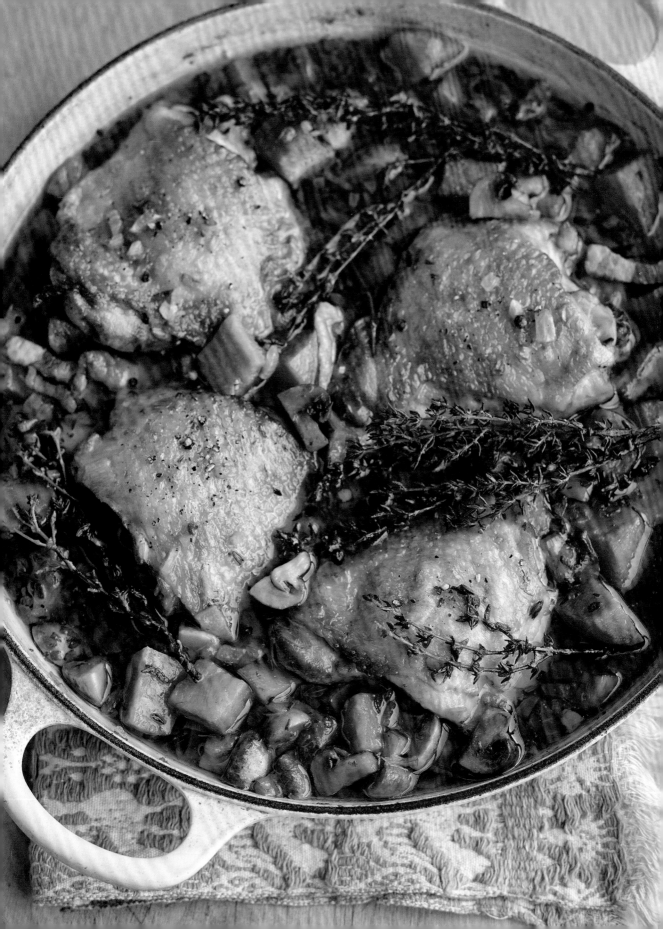

SERVES A FAMILY OF 4

PREP: 5 MINUTES
COOK: 30 MINUTES

This is a great supper dish that is full of flavour and very easy to make. The sauce creates a delicious broth, which is perfect paired with mashed potato or boiled rice.

Comforting
CHICKEN CASSEROLE

2 tablespoons olive oil

4 boneless chicken thighs with skin on

100g bacon lardons or chopped bacon

1 large onion, chopped

2 small sweet potatoes, peeled and cut into cubes

16 button mushrooms, cut into quarters

500ml Vegetable Stock (see page 248) or ½ low-salt vegetable stock cube ⚠ dissolved in 500ml boiling water

3 fresh thyme sprigs

1 Heat the oil in a heavy-based pan over a medium to high heat and fry the chicken, skin side down, until it becomes crispy. It will take about 5 minutes to get a lovely golden colour. Use a slotted spoon to remove the chicken pieces and set aside.

2 Pour away any excess fat and then, in the same pan, cook the bacon lardons and onions for about 5 minutes until they have taken on some colour.

3 Add the sweet potatoes and mushrooms and then return the chicken pieces to the pan, placing them on top, skin side up.

4 Pour over the stock until it just reaches the chicken skin, add the thyme and cover with a lid.

5 Leave to simmer very gently for about 10–15 minutes until the chicken is cooked through. The cooking time will depend on the size of the chicken pieces so do check by removing a piece of chicken and cutting into it with a sharp knife.

6 If you end up having more sauce than you'd like in the pan, simply strain into a clean saucepan, bring to the boil and reduce down by boiling it.

Optional Extras
You can add a few handfuls of cooked lentils or quinoa as they're both good sources of extra protein. Simply mix them in for the last 5 minutes of cooking.

Most families enjoy spaghetti bolognese as an easy and delicious supper dish and our version is rich and meaty and appeals to kids and adults alike. It works equally well with gluten-free spaghetti and pasta shapes and also tastes great served with a jacket potato. We always have a batch in our freezers because it seems to be universally liked, so is an easy supper if the children have friends over.

Meaty
BOLOGNESE SAUCE

2 tablespoons olive oil
500g beef mince
2 bacon rashers, chopped
1 onion, chopped
2 garlic cloves, crushed
1 large celery stick,
  sliced (optional)
400g tin chopped
  tomatoes
200ml Vegetable Stock
  (see page 248) or
  ½ low-salt vegetable
  stock cube (!)
  dissolved in 200ml
  boiling water
3 carrots, peeled
  and chopped
1 bay leaf
Freshly ground black
  pepper

1 Preheat the oven to 180°C/160°C fan/350°F/Gas mark 4.

2 Heat the oil in a large ovenproof dish over a medium to high heat. Add the beef mince and bacon bit by bit, allowing it to get some colour but being careful not to let it burn. It is best not to move the meat about too much initially, giving it a chance to take on a lovely brown colour.

3 Add the onion, stir and allow it to soften for a few minutes. Add the garlic and celery and cook for a further minute.

4 Add the tomatoes, stock and carrots and bring to a simmer. Drop in the bay leaf.

5 Put on a lid and pop it into the oven for 1½ hours, giving it a quick stir every 30 minutes. Don't skimp on the cooking time – this dish really needs it to allow the meat to become very tender and to create a thick, tasty sauce.

6 Remove the bay leaf and season to taste before serving.

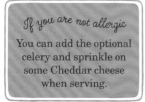

If you are not allergic
You can add the optional celery and sprinkle on some Cheddar cheese when serving.

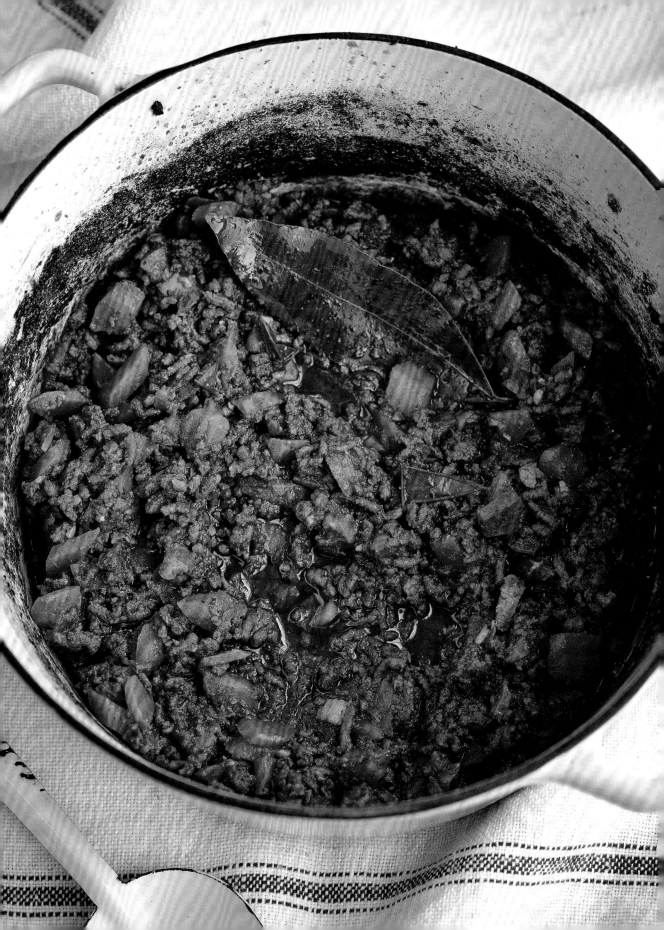

SERVES A FAMILY OF 4

PREP: 5 MINUTES
COOK: 1¼ HOURS

This is another family classic, but our version has no chilli in it, just lots of lovely aromatic earthy flavours and delicious kidney beans. Of course you can add chilli afterwards or serve with some jalapeño peppers if you like a little heat. This is a big hit with Casper and his friends and makes a really fun meal if you prepare cucumbers, tomatoes, Guacamole (see page 133) and taco shells so the kids can get stuck in and help themselves to a feast. Or simply serve with some steamed rice and peas.

Chilli
CON CARNE

1 tablespoon olive oil
500g beef mince
¼ small onion, chopped
1 small red pepper,
  deseeded and chopped
1 small yellow pepper,
  deseeded and chopped
1 teaspoon ground cumin
1 teaspoon ground
  coriander
2 teaspoons cumin seeds
400g tin kidney beans,
  drained and rinsed
400g tin chopped
  tomatoes
250ml water

1 Preheat the oven to 180°C/160°C fan/350°F/Gas mark 4.

2 Heat the oil in a heavy-based ovenproof pan over a medium to high heat. Add the mince, bit by bit, allowing it to get some colour but being careful not to let it burn. It is best not to move it about too much initially, giving it a chance to take on a lovely brown colour.

3 Fry the onion and peppers for a couple of minutes, allowing them to soften a little.

4 Add the ground cumin, coriander and cumin seeds and then stir well.

5 Add the kidney beans, chopped tomatoes and water and give a stir to make sure everything is combined.

6 Transfer the pan to the oven for 1½ hours, stirring every 30 minutes. Skim off any excess fat before serving.

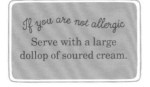

If you are not allergic
Serve with a large
dollop of soured cream.

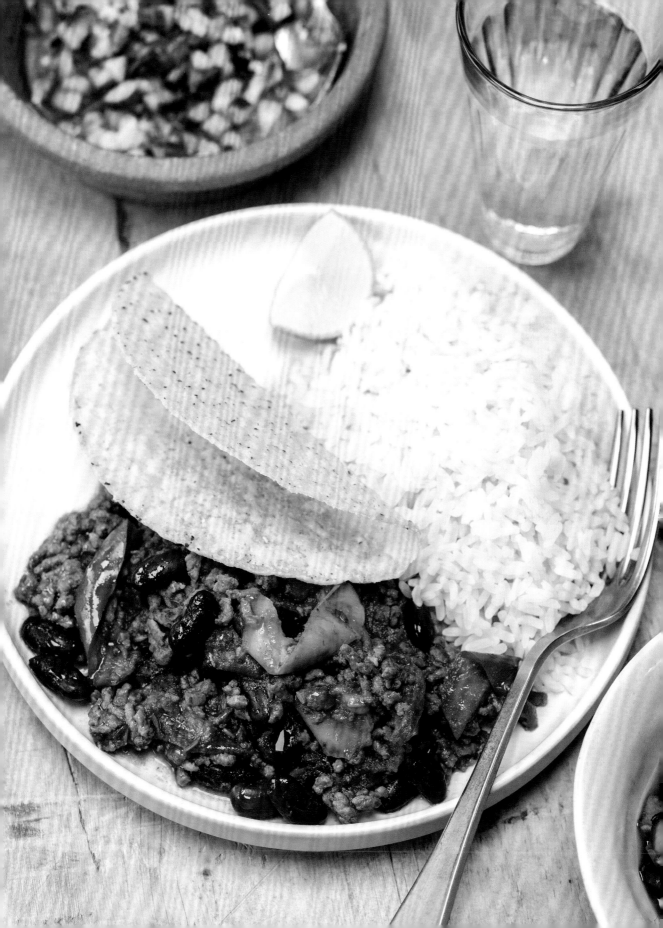

SERVES A FAMILY OF 4

PREP: 5 MINUTES
COOK: 1¼ HOURS

This is an easy beef casserole that is quick to prepare and is a tasty recipe for younger and older kids alike. It must be allowed a long, slow cook to make the meat deliciously tender so don't be tempted to take it out of the oven early. This is a lovely warming dish for the autumn and winter and is great served with mashed or jacket potatoes.

One-Pot
BEEF STEW

1 tablespoon olive oil
800g stewing beef, chopped
½ small onion, chopped
2 leeks, chopped
1 swede, peeled and chopped
2 carrots, peeled and chopped
1 celery stick, chopped (optional)
500ml water

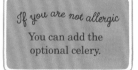

If you are not allergic
You can add the optional celery.

1 Preheat the oven to 180°C/160°C fan/350°F/Gas mark 4.

2 Heat the oil in a heavy-based, ovenproof pan or casserole over a medium to high heat and brown the beef. Do this in batches if you need to as overcrowding the pan will stop the meat browning. You are looking for a little colour on all the pieces of meat and this will take a good few minutes without moving the meat about too much. This browning process helps add a lovely rich taste to the dish.

3 Add the onion, stir well and cook for a couple of minutes until it has softened a little.

4 Add the leeks, swede, carrots, celery and water and then bring to a simmer.

5 Cover with a lid and place in the oven for 1½ hours, stirring occasionally. Add a little extra water if needed. Check the meat is lovely and tender before serving.

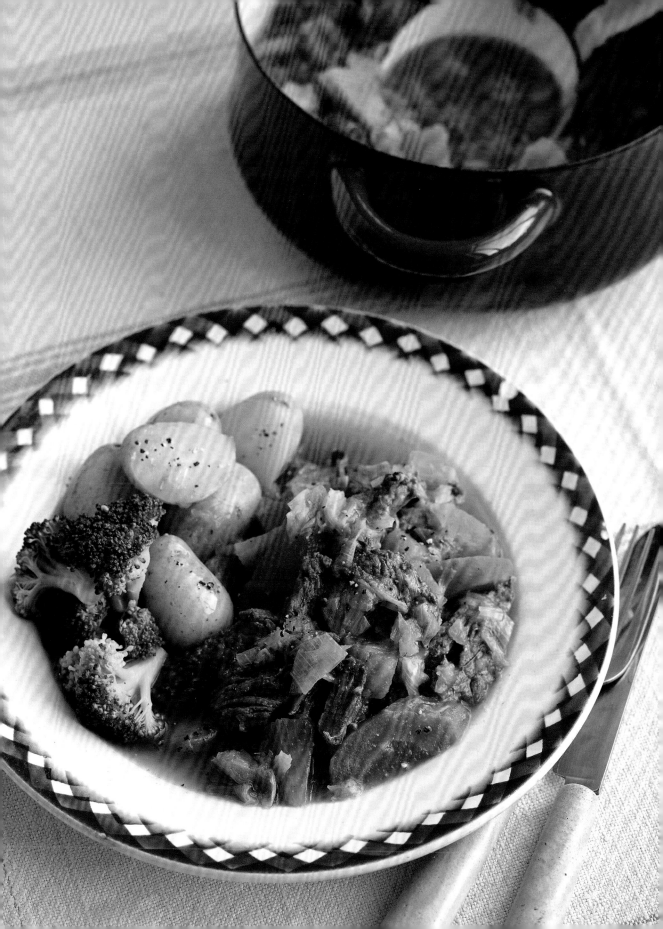

PREP: 5 MINUTES
COOK: 1¼ HOURS

Goulash is a Hungarian stew flavoured with paprika, which is a wonderfully earthy spice that gives a lovely colour and richness to the dish. This recipe is particularly tasty when made with sweet smoked paprika, which is easy to find in supermarkets, but beware that some varieties of paprika can be hot. There is only a little paprika in this recipe so it is mild and not overpowering. Don't be tempted to put the peppers in at the beginning as they will cook down and break up in the stew. We like this served with mash and green beans.

Beef GOULASH

1 teaspoon olive oil
500g stewing beef, chopped
2 onions, sliced
2 garlic cloves, crushed
½ level tablespoon sweet smoked paprika
2 x 400g tins chopped tomatoes
250ml water
1 bay leaf
2 red peppers, deseeded and sliced

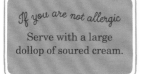

If you are not allergic
Serve with a large dollop of soured cream.

1 Preheat the oven to 180°C/160°C fan/350°F/Gas mark 4.

2 Heat the oil in a heavy-based, ovenproof pan or casserole over a medium to high heat and brown the beef. Do this in batches if you need to and ideally without moving the meat about too much. This will take about 5 minutes and you are looking for a little colour on all the pieces of meat, which will help give a lovely rich taste to the dish.

3 Add the onions and garlic, stir through and cook for a few minutes until they have begun to soften.

4 Add the paprika and stir and then add the tomatoes and water. Bring to a simmer.

5 Add the bay leaf, cover with a lid and place in the oven for 1 hour. It will need this length of time to allow the meat to become really tender and soft.

6 Remove from the oven and add the peppers and a touch more water if too much of the liquid has evaporated. Pop back in the oven to cook for a further 30 minutes. You are looking for a nice thick sauce to coat the meat.

7 Remove the bay leaf before serving.

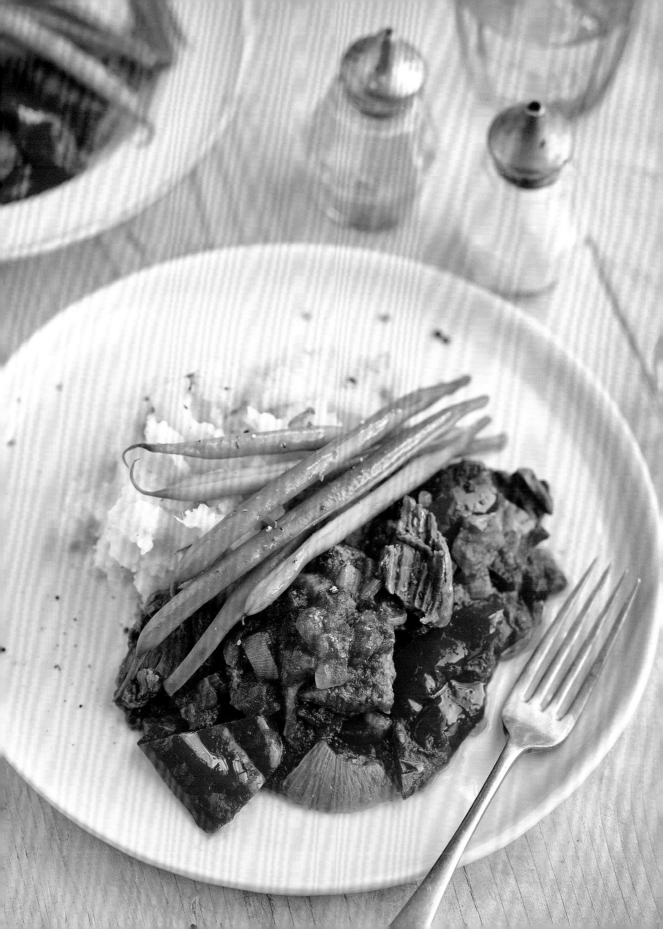

This is a traditional Moroccan dish. Our version is mildly flavoured so not overpowering for younger children. The sauce is quite thick, making this is a wonderfully comforting dish, ideally served with boiled rice and green vegetables or salad leaves. Lamb is often expensive but by using a cheaper cut like neck fillet you get loads of flavour. It is essential that you give this dish a long, slow cook so that the meat becomes really tender to the point that it just melts in the mouth. This is always a popular option with Isabelle and Zara.

Moroccan Spiced
LAMB TAGINE

½ tablespoon olive oil

450g lamb neck fillet, chopped into chunks

1 large onion, chopped

1 garlic clove, crushed

1 teaspoon ground cumin

1 teaspoon ground coriander

¼ teaspoon ground cinnamon

400g tin chopped tomatoes

400g tin chickpeas, drained and rinsed

150g (or a good handful) dried apricots, cut in half

30g raisins

1 tablespoon runny honey

350ml water

Freshly ground black pepper

1 Preheat the oven to 180°C/160°C fan/350°F/Gas mark 4.

2 Heat the oil in a heavy-based, ovenproof pan or casserole over a medium to high heat and brown the meat. Cook in batches if necessary. You are looking for a little colour on all the pieces of meat and this will take a good few minutes without moving the meat about too much in the pan.

3 Add the onion and cook for a few minutes until it has begun to soften. Add the garlic and spices and stir for a further minute.

4 Add the chopped tomatoes, chickpeas, apricots, raisins, honey and water. Bring to a simmer, cover with a lid and transfer to the oven for 1½–2 hours until the lamb becomes lovely and tender.

5 Stir occasionally during the cooking process and if it looks like a lot of the juice has evaporated, add a little more water if needed. You are looking for the initial liquid to be reduced by about half to make a lovely thick sauce. Season to taste.

If you are not allergic
This dish also goes really well with wholemeal couscous.

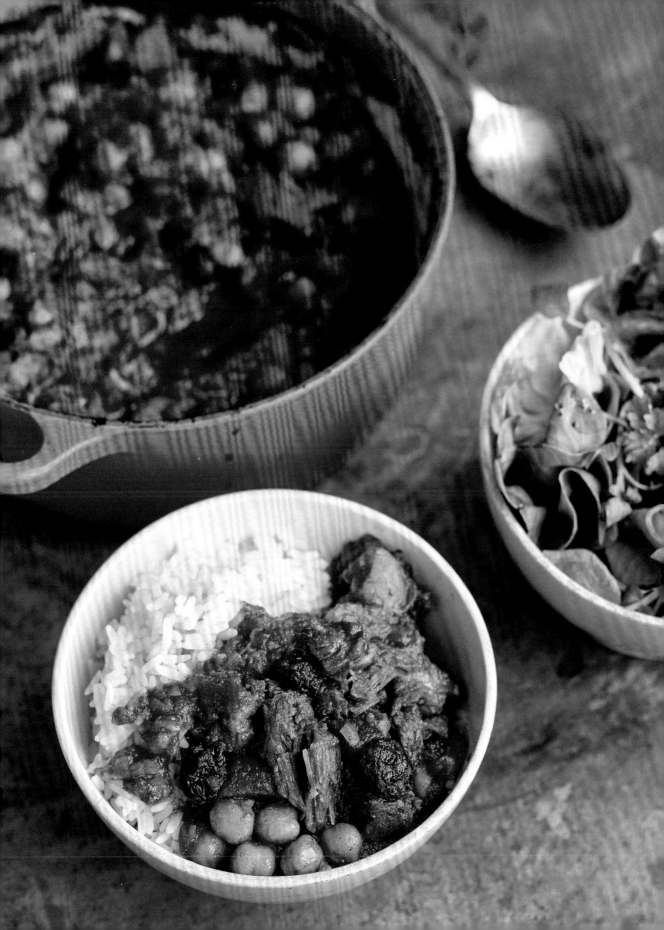

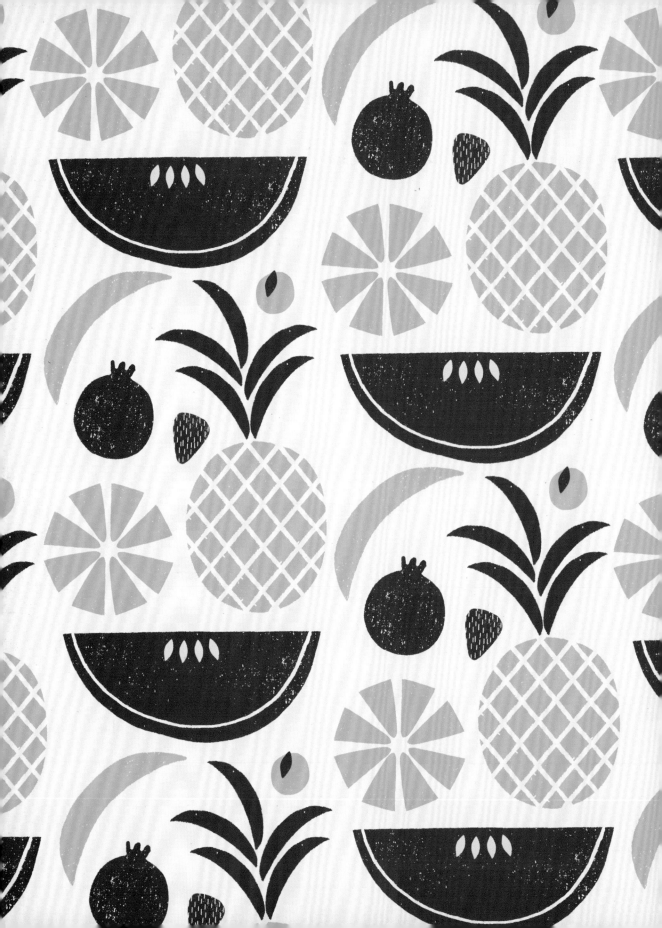

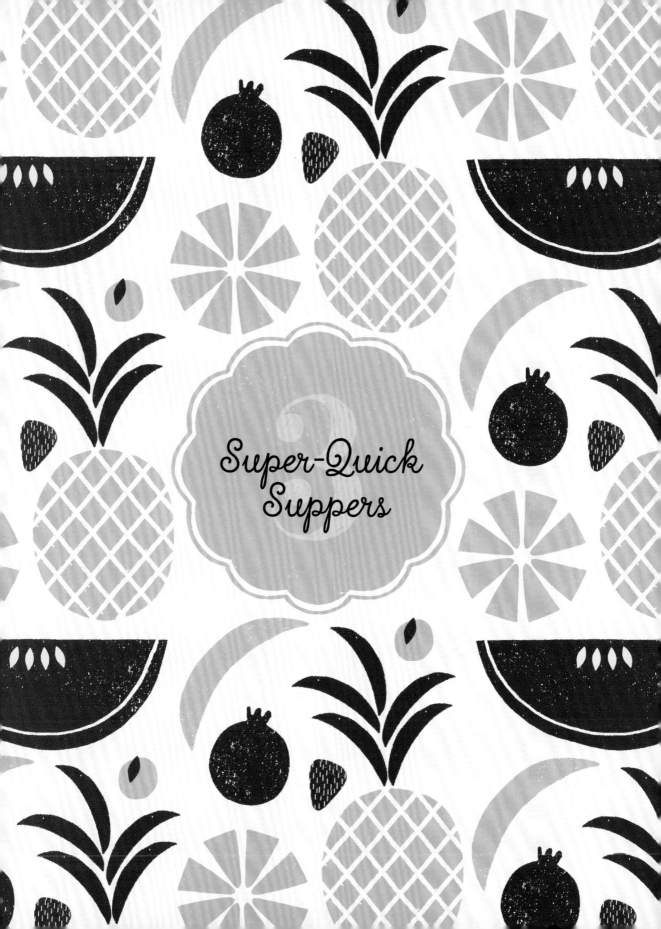

Super-Quick
Suppers

There's nothing worse than coming home late after a busy day, with the children moaning they're hungry and knowing you won't have dinner on the table for ages. We all have so much on day-to-day, so it's helpful to have a range of nutritious meals on hand that you know you can rustle up quickly. The recipes in this section are both quick to prepare and quick to cook, so you can make a meal from scratch in minutes (even if your knife skills leave something to be desired). We cook these recipes at home all the time because they are so easy and fast and the children really love them.

We tend to cook separately for our kids on school nights, so these recipes are all quick mid-week kids' suppers designed to serve two children but you can, of course, increase the portions to feed more children or indeed the whole family.

All our children love the Vietnamese Rice Noodle Soup (see page 81), which we often have when we've had a roast chicken over the weekend so we can use up the leftovers. Izzy is also a big fan of the Pork Meatballs (see page 90). Casper loves Skate with Capers (see page 72) – in fact, he loves it so much that he is now on first name terms with Tommy at the fish counter!

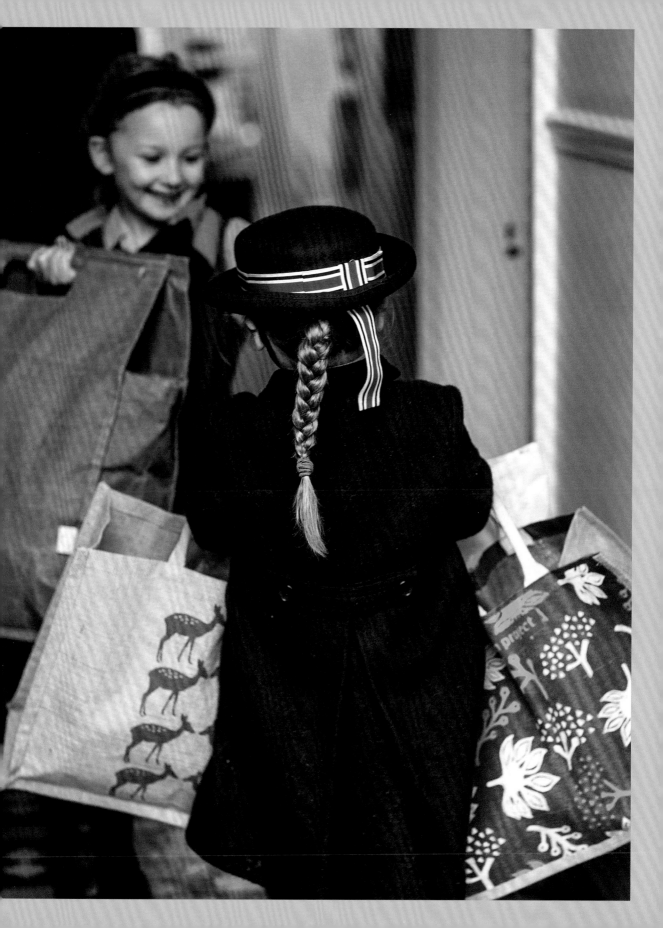

This is a classic combination of Mediterranean flavours. Some types of fish are over-exploited and it is worth making sure your cod is from a sustainable source. If you prefer, this recipe is equally delicious with other firm white fish such as coley, pollock, pouting or tilapia. Turn this into a really easy meal for the whole family by doubling the quantities and using adult-sized fish portions. Delicious served with broccoli and fine green beans.

ROASTED COD
with Potatoes, Tomato and Olives

250g small new potatoes
1 tablespoon olive oil
12 cherry tomatoes, halved
4 garlic cloves, peeled and left whole
2 x 60g skinless filleted firm white fish of your choice
8 pitted olives, green or black (buy a full-flavour olive such as Kalamata)
25ml water
Handful fresh basil leaves
Freshly ground black pepper

1 Preheat the oven to 220°C/200°C fan/425°F/Gas mark 7.

2 Put the potatoes in a saucepan, cover with cold water and bring to a simmer. Cook until they feel just tender, then drain and slice them in half.

3 Put the oil, cherry tomatoes, garlic and potatoes in a deep-sided baking tray and cook in the oven for 10 minutes.

4 Remove the tray from the oven and add the cod, olives and water. Return the tray to the oven and cook for a further 5–10 minutes or until the cod is cooked through.

5 Sprinkle with basil leaves and season to taste before serving.

VARIATION
Follow the recipe as above, replacing the cod with 1 sliced chicken breast at step 4.

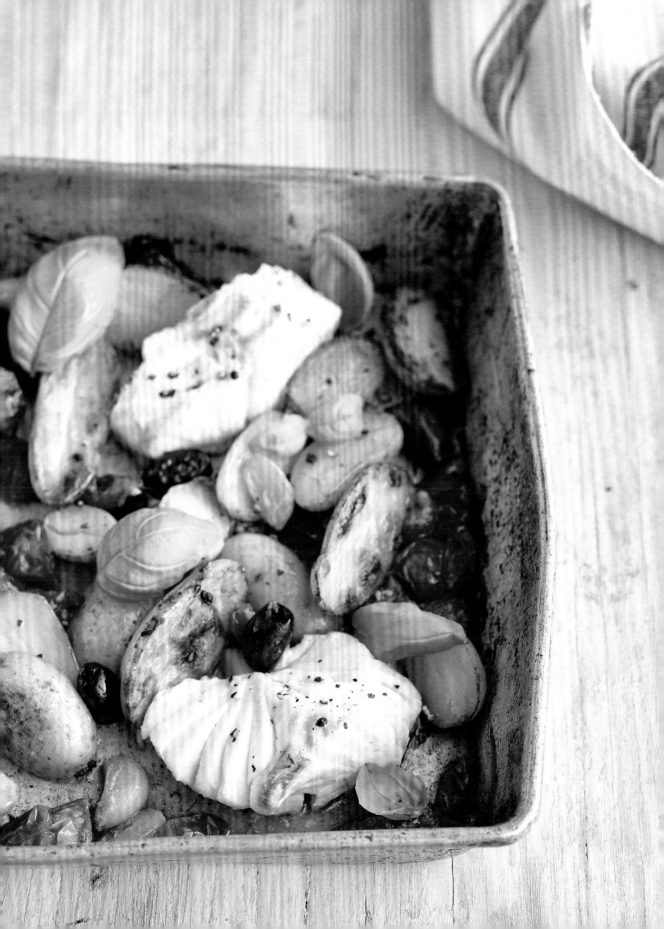

SERVES 2 CHILDREN

PREP: 5 MINUTES
COOK: 15 MINUTES

This method of steaming fish in a little parcel is very easy and can be used for other types of fish according to preference. The most important thing is that the parcel is tightly shut so the steam inside cooks the fish beautifully, rather than escaping. You can make the parcel up to a day ahead and leave in the fridge until you are ready to cook. Serve with boiled new potatoes and courgettes.

SALMON WITH TOMATO
and Basil Cooked in a Parcel

Drizzle of olive oil
2 x 60g portions of
   salmon, skin removed
4 lemon slices
8 cherry tomatoes,
   sliced in half
12 large fresh basil
   leaves, roughly torn
Freshly ground black
   pepper

1 Preheat the oven to 220°C/200°C fan/425°F/Gas mark 7.

2 Lay out a piece of baking paper, about 40 x 40cm, on a baking tray and drizzle one side with a little oil.

3 Sandwich each piece of salmon between 2 slices of lemon and place on the oiled baking paper.

4 Scatter the tomatoes and basil leaves around the fish and season with black pepper.

5 Fold over the baking paper and wrap the parcel tightly on all sides so no steam can escape.

6 Cook for 10–15 minutes, depending on the thickness of the fish. If the fish is not cooked when you remove from the oven, simply wrap the paper up again and pop back in the oven for a few more minutes until it is cooked through.

VARIATION
Follow the recipe as above, replacing the salmon with 2 small chicken breasts at step 3.

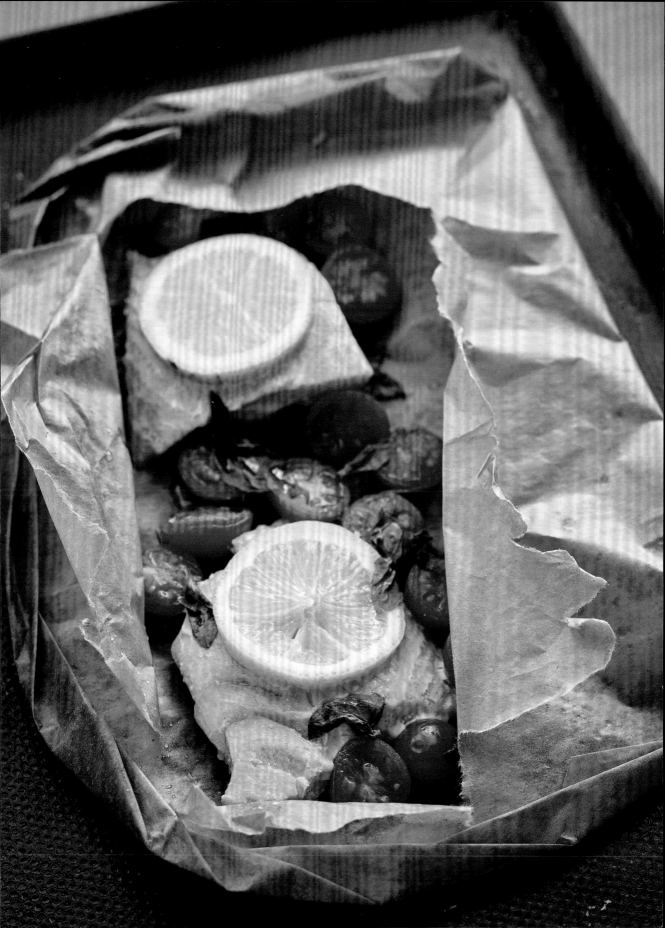

PREP: 5 MINUTES
COOK: 5 MINUTES

This dish is a really simple and quick way to cook salmon and vegetables in one go, especially as you can pop it in the microwave. Some kids like it with lots of the cooking juice as a sauce, and some just like a drizzle on top. This is lovely served with some simply boiled basmati rice.

SALMON
with Orange and Ginger

2 x 60g portions
    of salmon
2 large broccoli florets,
    cut into very small
    pieces
Handful frozen peas
1 teaspoon grated
    or finely chopped
    fresh ginger
Juice of 2 oranges or
    150ml orange juice
    from a carton
Orange zest (optional)

1 Place the portions of fish, vegetables and ginger in a small saucepan and pour over the orange juice, making sure all the ingredients are covered.

2 Bring to a gentle simmer and poach for 5 minutes. Alternatively, pop all the ingredients in a microwavable bowl, cover with clingfilm and microwave on high for 3–5 minutes.

3 Check the fish is cooked through before serving and sprinkle over the orange zest, if using.

> *If you are not allergic*
> This goes well with
> wholemeal couscous.

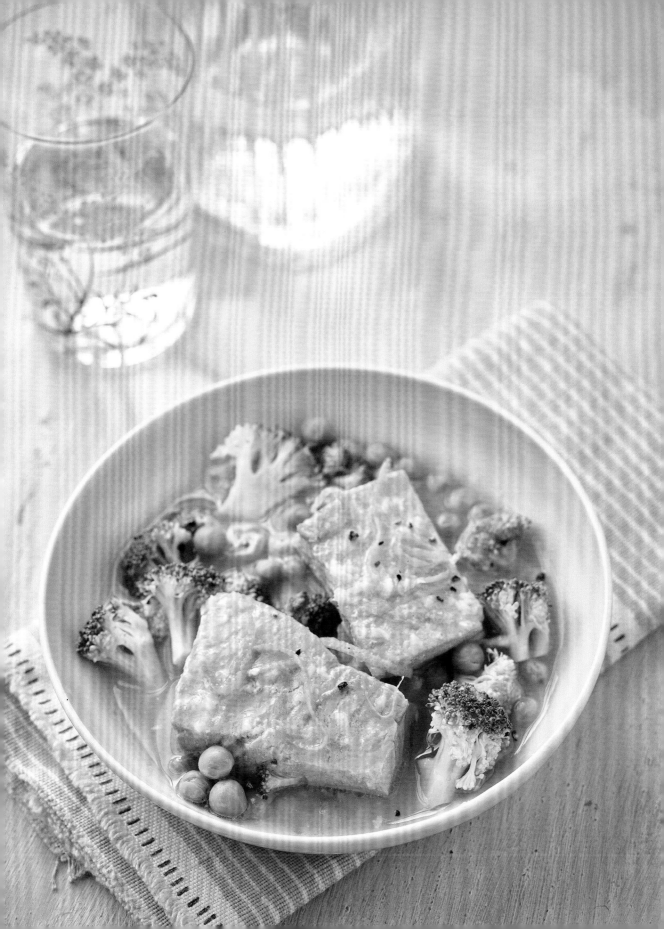

PREP: 5 MINUTES
COOK: 10 MINUTES

Skate is a great fish to serve children as it has no bones – just a piece of cartilage that is very easy to remove, leaving plenty of soft, white fish. Skate with capers is a classic combination but this recipe works just as well with ray wing which is similar and easier to get hold of. This recipe is also good just with a squeeze of lemon juice and a bit of chopped parsley if your children wrinkle their noses at the idea of capers. Casper likes this best served with Mashed Potato (see page 182) or Potato Wedges (see page 184) and peas.

SKATE *with Capers*

2 teaspoons olive oil
200g piece of skate
 or ray wing
1 tablespoon dairy-free
 sunflower spread
 (optional)
1 teaspoon capers
 (optional)
Good squeeze of
 lemon juice

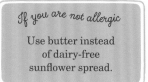

If you are not allergic

Use butter instead
of dairy-free
sunflower spread.

1 Heat a little oil in a frying pan and cook the skate on both sides over a medium to low heat for about 6 minutes until it is cooked through.

2 Remove the fish and take off the flesh with a fork ready to serve on to the plates – it should come away very easily on both sides from the single piece of cartilage in the middle. If you do break it, don't worry, but try to avoid putting any broken bits of cartilage on the plate.

3 Add a little more oil or sunflower spread to the pan, add the capers and lemon juice just for a few moments to warm through and then pour over the fish.

Optional Extras
Sprinkle with a small handful of chopped fresh parsley before serving.

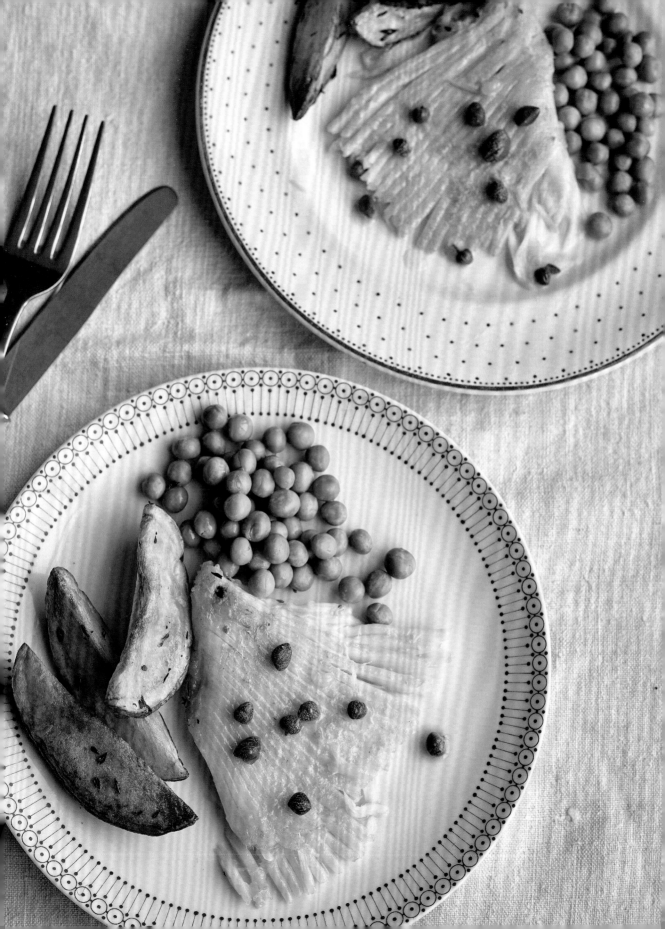

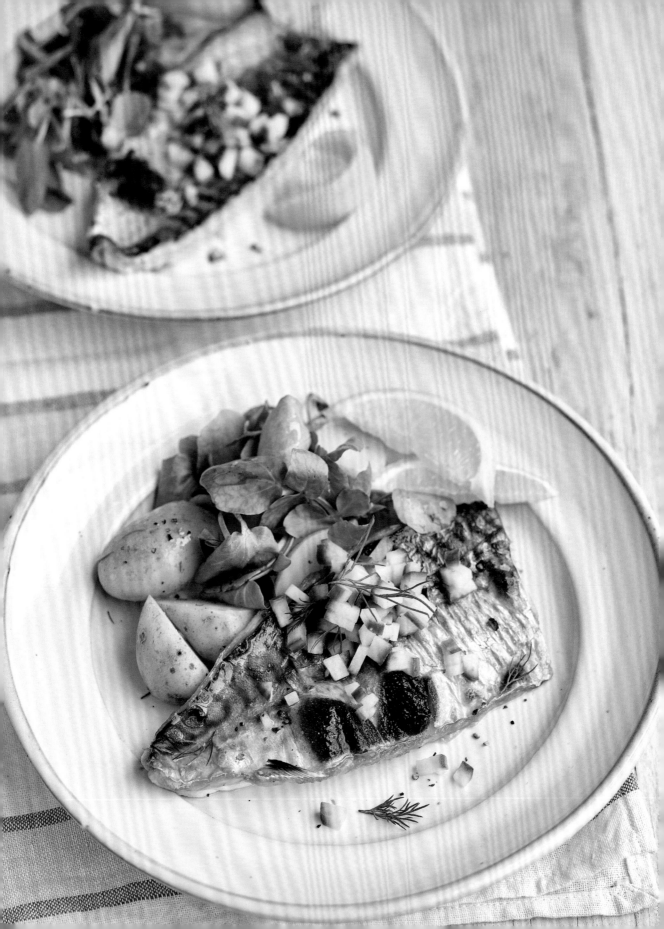

PREP: 10 MINUTES
COOK: 10 MINUTES

As mackerel is an oily fish, it is great served with something fresh, so cucumber is the perfect addition. This is a lovely light summer dish and delicious with new potatoes and a crisp green salad. You can cook a whole fish if you are confident separating the fish bones, otherwise just buy fillets. This is a popular recipe with both our families.

GRILLED MACKEREL
with Lemon and Cucumber

2 mackerel fillets
Olive oil, for drizzling
Squeeze of lemon juice
¼ cucumber, cut into small cubes
A few sprigs of fresh dill (or parsley if you prefer), chopped

1 Use your fingers to feel along the flesh of the mackerel fillet to check for bones, just in case any have been missed in the filleting process. If there are any, simply remove with a pair of kitchen tweezers.

2 Preheat the grill to a medium to high heat.

3 Drizzle a little olive oil over the mackerel and then cook under the hot grill for about 5 minutes until cooked through. Turning the fish over halfway through the cooking process to grill the skin will make it lovely and crispy.

4 Transfer the mackerel to 2 plates. Squeeze the lemon juice over the top and then sprinkle with cucumber and dill before serving.

PREP: 5 MINUTES
COOK: 5 MINUTES

This is such a simple meal and great for younger kids as it is very plain. You can easily serve it with just a squeeze of lemon or, as the recipe suggests, make a little parsley salsa to go on top. If you want some variety this recipe is also lovely with plaice – but no matter what fish you use it is great and Zara and Izzy particularly like it with a side of chips and garden peas. If your child is not a fish eater then this parsley salsa is also really good with a plain cooked chicken breast.

PAN-FRIED LEMON SOLE
with Parsley Salsa

Olive oil, for drizzling
2 small lemon sole fillets
  or 1 large fillet

Parsley salsa
Juice of ½ lemon
Small handful fresh
  parsley, chopped
1 tablespoon olive oil
½ small garlic clove
2 cornichons
½ teaspoon capers
Freshly ground black
  pepper
Lemon zest (optional)

1 Heat the oil in a pan, add the lemon sole fillets, skin side down, and pan fry gently over a medium to low heat until the flesh is cooked through. This should take about 5 minutes.

2 Put all the salsa ingredients in a blender and blitz until they are all well combined.

3 Drizzle the salsa over the cooked fish before serving and sprinkle over the lemon zest, if using.

VARIATION
Follow the recipe above, replacing the sole with 1 butterflied and flattened chicken breast at step 1.

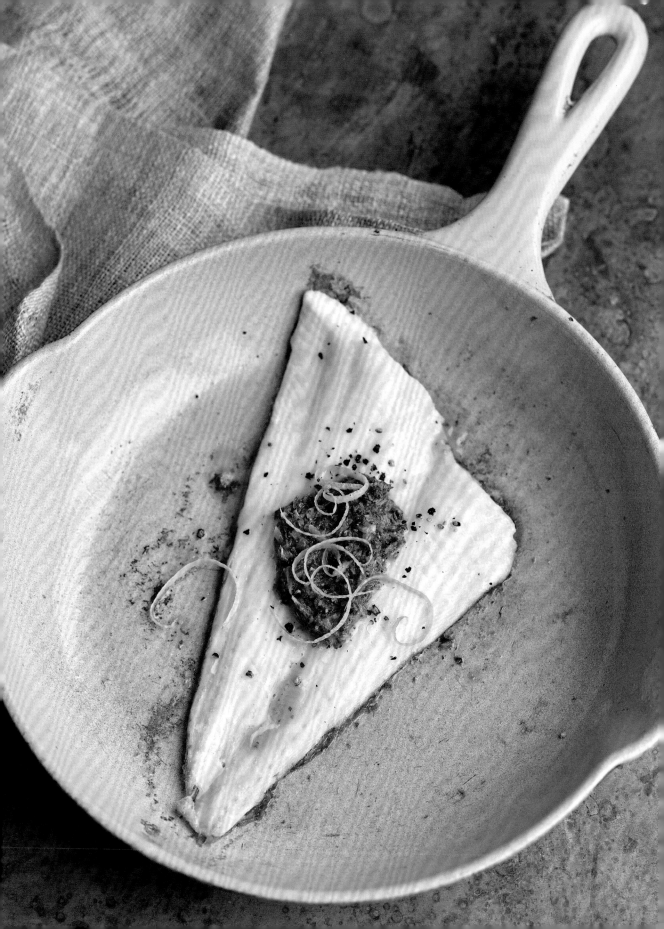

SERVES **2** CHILDREN

PREP: 10 MINUTES
COOK: NONE

A Niçoise salad will usually be served with a boiled egg but is just as delicious without. This is a classic recipe from the south of France and is a lovely meal to serve in the summer. It is very quick and easy to assemble, especially if you use tinned tuna. While fresh tuna is a great source of Omega-3 fatty acids, tinned tuna is not due to the canning process. If you are using tinned tuna, it is better to buy tuna tinned in olive oil as tuna in brine contains a lot of salt. Finally, remember to try to buy line-caught tuna.

Eggless NIÇOISE SALAD

1 little gem lettuce, leaves separated and washed
¼ cucumber, sliced
2 tomatoes, quartered or cut into chunks
Large handful fine green beans, boiled and then plunged into cold water to chill quickly
200g new potatoes, cooked and cooled
80g tuna (best fresh, seared on both sides or tinned in olive oil)
12 pitted black or green olives (a flavoursome variety like Kalamata is best)

Dressing
Juice of ½ lemon
2 tablespoons olive oil

1 Arrange a layer of lettuce on two plates and then top with the cucumber, tomatoes, beans, potatoes and tuna. Finally, scatter over the olives.

2 Combine the oil and lemon juice in a small bowl or jar. Pour the dressing over the top to serve or serve it on the side.

VARIATION
Substitute the tuna with 1 chicken breast, cut into thin strips and then pan-fried for 5–6 minutes until cooked.

> *If you are not allergic*
> A hard-boiled egg cut into quarters can be added.

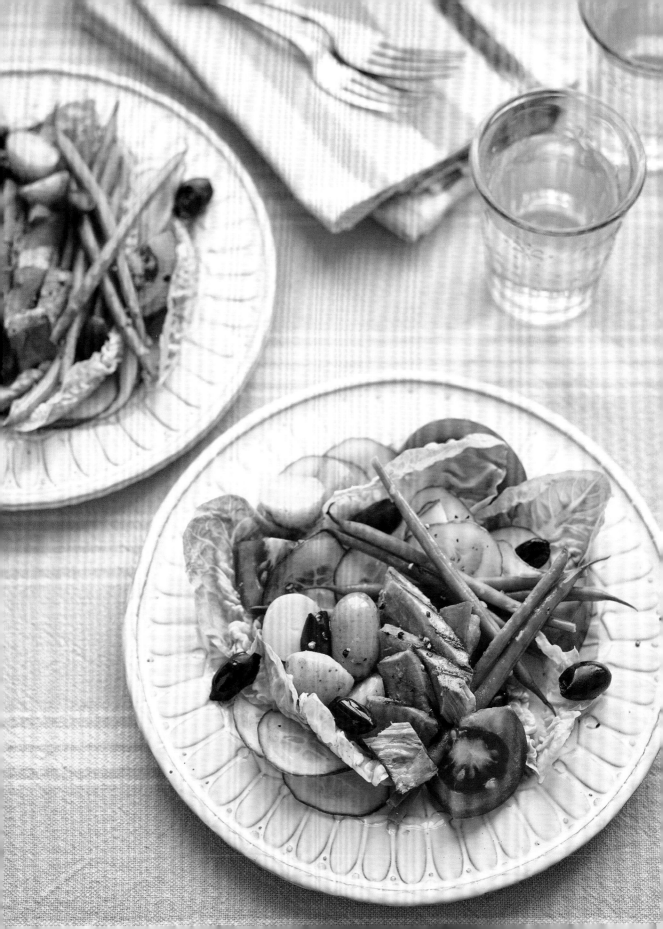

SERVES 2 CHILDREN

PREP: 10 MINUTES
COOK: 5 MINUTES

This is a fun, casual supper dish that takes moments to assemble and the kids absolutely love it. If children are fussy eaters, getting them involved in assembling their own food and eating with their fingers is a way of keeping mealtimes fun and encouraging little ones to join in and enjoy their food.

Chilli NACHOS

300g portion Chilli Con Carne (see page 54)
4 handfuls plain, unsalted corn chips ⚠
8 tablespoons guacamole ⚠ (or make your own, see page 133)
4 tomatoes, chopped into chunks
1 small cucumber, chopped into chunks
A few jalapeño peppers from a jar (optional)

1 Reheat the Chilli Con Carne if necessary.

2 Arrange a layer of corn chips on two plates and top with the Chilli Con Carne, guacamole, tomatoes, cucumber and jalapeño peppers, if using.

3 Alternatively, serve all components in separate bowls for everyone to help themselves to and make up their own nacho dish.

> *If you are not allergic*
> Add a good sprinkle of cheese on top or a generous dollop of soured cream.

PREP: 10 MINUTES
COOK: 15 MINUTES

We travelled in Vietnam together when we were students and really enjoyed the cuisine. This recipe is inspired by some of the lovely street food we ate on our travels. Casper and Cammie love eating these steaming bowls of noodles with Chinese spoons and chopsticks. For more advanced palates add a little chopped chilli. We regularly make this when we've had leftover roast chicken to use up. Fresh rice noodles are available from most major supermarkets.

Vietnamese RICE NOODLE SOUP

1 teaspoon olive oil

2 teaspoons chopped onion

3 tablespoons Homemade Southeast Asian Blend (see page 251)

300ml fresh Chicken Stock (see page 250) or ½ low-salt vegetable stock cube ❗ dissolved in 300ml boiling water

1 courgette, quartered lengthways and chopped into small chunks

6 baby sweetcorn, chopped into rounds

100g leftover roast chicken or cooked chicken breast, shredded

150g fresh rice noodles

6 cherry tomatoes, halved

Lime wedges, for squeezing

Handful fresh coriander, chopped

Small handful fresh mint leaves, finely chopped

A few Thai basil leaves, roughly torn (optional)

1 Heat the oil in a large saucepan over a high heat. Fry the onion and Southeast Asian Blend for a few minutes and then add the stock and bring it to a simmer.

2 Add the courgette and sweetcorn and cook for a few more minutes until the vegetables start to become tender.

3 Add the chicken, noodles and tomatoes and then simmer for a few more minutes.

4 Ladle the soup into bowls, allow to cool a little and serve with a wedge of lime and some fresh chopped coriander, mint and basil as a garnish.

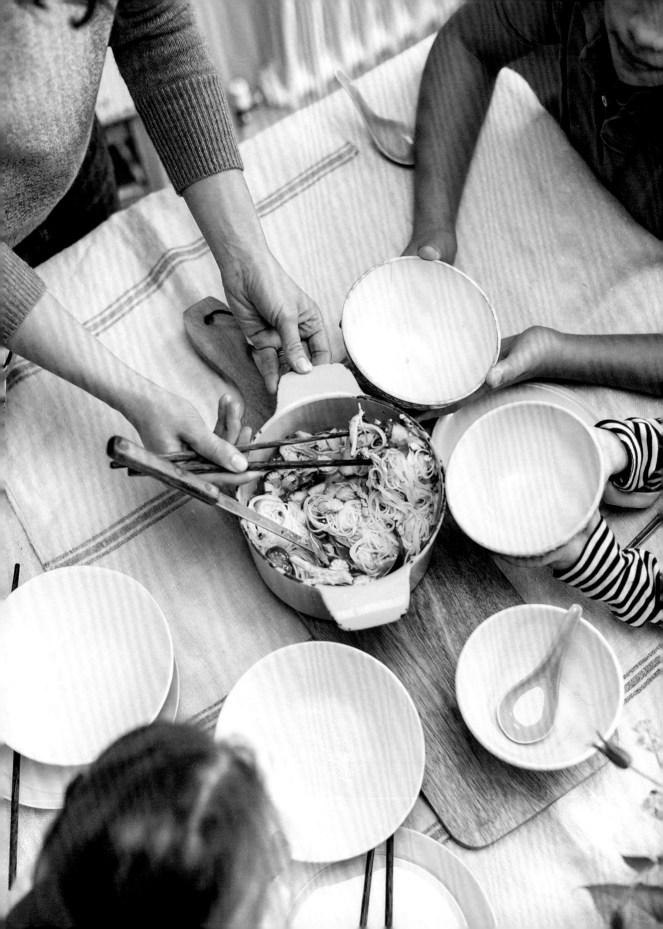

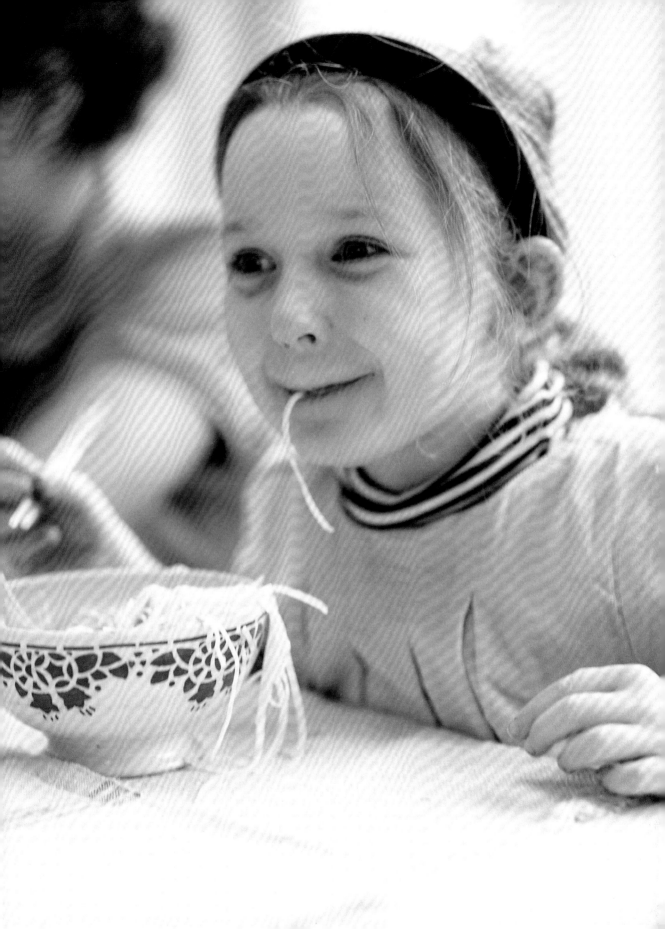

PREP: 10 MINUTES
COOK: NONE

This is great for using up any leftover roast chicken or you can cook a piece of chicken especially for it. Chicken and mango are always a great combination for a salad and it makes a lovely fresh and fruity meal that really appeals to kids. It is a good idea to expose children to a variety of flavours early on so that they are open to eating a range of different foods later on in life. Both our families eat this a lot in the summer.

Fresh and Sweet
CHICKEN AND MANGO SALAD

1 cooked chicken breast (or equivalent amount of leftover roast chicken), chilled and shredded

1 mango, skin removed, stoned and diced

A few very thin slices of red onion

¼ cucumber, cut into small cubes

10 fresh mint leaves, finely sliced

Handful fresh coriander leaves (you can use flat-leaf parsley instead if you prefer), chopped

1 little gem lettuce, shredded

Freshly ground black pepper

Dressing
Juice of 1 lime
1 tablespoon olive oil

1 Combine all the salad ingredients in a bowl and mix well.

2 Mix the dressing ingredients in another bowl and add to the salad, coating well before serving.

> *If you are not allergic*
> Gently toast some sesame seeds to sprinkle on the top and add a little sesame oil to the dressing.

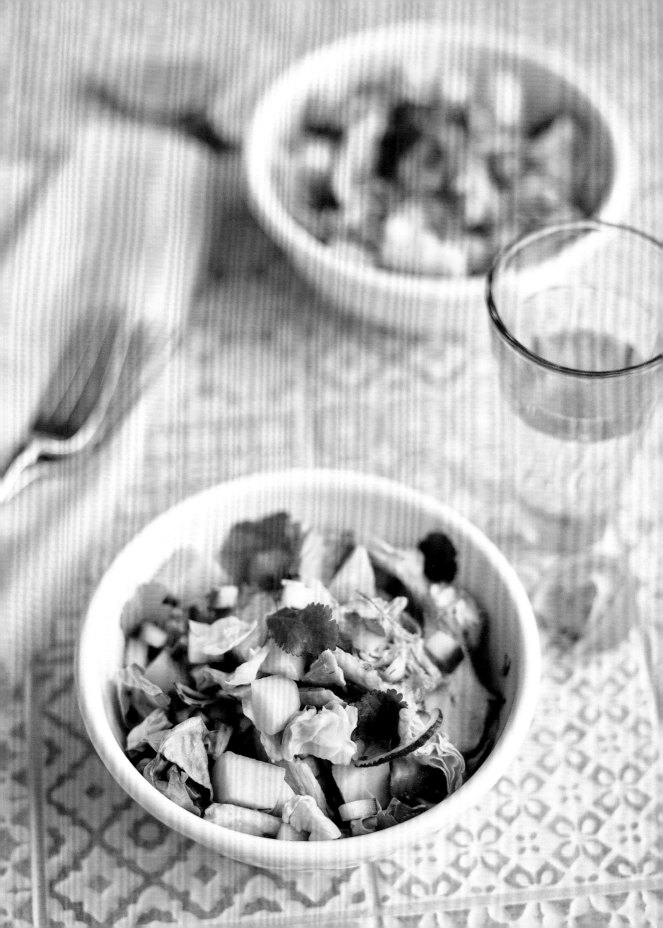

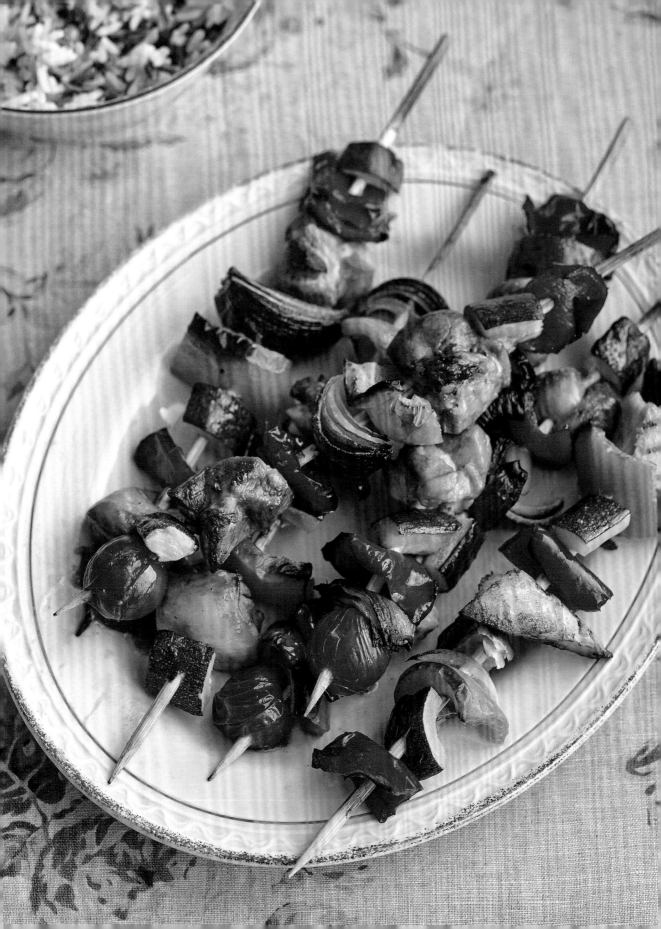

PREP: 10 MINUTES
COOK: 10 MINUTES

These are very easy to make, look really good and kids love the fact they can pick the kebabs up with their fingers – so they're often a hit with fussy eaters. The kebabs are equally tasty cooked under the grill, in your oven or on the barbecue and so simple to prepare in advance if you are entertaining; just assemble, cover and pop in the fridge the day before. If you use chicken thigh meat you will get a better flavour and it is less expensive than other cuts. However, chicken breast or even turkey will work just as well. Zara and Isabelle love these kebabs served with long grain and wild rice.

Colourful CHICKEN AND VEG KEBABS

Bamboo or metal skewers
4 skinless and boneless
   chicken thigh fillets, cut
   into bite-size pieces
1 courgette, sliced and
   halved if very large
1 small red pepper,
   deseeded and chopped
1 small yellow pepper,
   deseeded and chopped
1 small green pepper,
   deseeded and chopped
½ small red onion, cut
   into bite-size pieces
16 cherry tomatoes,
   left whole
1 tablespoon olive oil

1 If using bamboo rather than metal skewers, soak them in water for 30 minutes to stop them burning under the grill.

2 Toss the meat and vegetables in a bowl with a little oil so everything is lightly coated.

3 Thread the meat and vegetables onto the skewers. Preheat the grill to a medium to high heat.

4 Grill the kebabs under the hot grill for about 5–10 minutes depending on how large the chunks of meat are. These can also be cooked in a preheated oven at 220°C/200°C fan/425°F/Gas mark 7 for about 10 minutes or on a hot barbecue or griddle pan.

5 Check the chicken is cooked through before serving.

SERVES 2 CHILDREN

PREP: 15 MINUTES,
PLUS MARINATING
COOK: 10 MINUTES

Chicken with lemon and garlic is a lovely combination. This recipe also works well with small pieces of chicken threaded onto a skewer to make a kebab – just reduce the cooking time slightly. This light dish, perfect for a barbecue, is lovely served with long grain rice and our Tomato Salsa (see page 137).

Summer LEMON CHICKEN

2 skinless chicken thigh
   fillets, flattened out
2 garlic cloves, crushed
Juice of 1 lemon
1 teaspoon olive oil
Good handful fresh
   parsley, chopped

1 Preheat oven to 220°C/200°C fan/425°F/Gas mark 7.

2 Place all the ingredients in a bowl, mix together and leave to marinate for 10 minutes. Don't be tempted to marinate for much longer as the acid in the lemon juice will start to make the meat a bit mushy.

3 Take the chicken pieces, place on a baking tray and cook in the oven for about 10 minutes. Check the chicken is cooked through before serving.

SERVES
2
CHILDREN

PREP: 5 MINUTES
COOK: 10 MINUTES

This is a really easy recipe that takes just moments to pull together. As an added bonus figs are an excellent additional source of calcium. Ideal for a light bite or starter, this dish is great eaten cold but it's even better assembled and then baked in the oven.

FIGS
with Parma Ham

4 fresh figs
4 Parma ham
   or prosciutto
   ham slices
½ tablespoon
   runny honey
Olive oil, for drizzling
Balsamic vinegar,
   for drizzling
Freshly ground black
   pepper

1 Slice open the figs by making a cross on the top, being careful not to actually cut them into quarters, and squeeze them slightly at the base to open them up.

2 Drape a piece of ham over each fig.

3 Drizzle with a little honey, olive oil and balsamic vinegar.

4 Serve cold or pop in an oven preheated to 200°C/180°C fan/400°F/Gas mark 6 for 10 minutes or until the ham crisps up.

5 Season with a little pepper to taste.

VARIATION
Simply drape Parma ham slices over slices of honeydew melon instead.

If you are not allergic
Fill the centre of the fig with a little cream cheese or soft goat's cheese before you drape over the ham.

Everyone loves meatballs and these are extra special as the apple makes them really moist and gives them a hint of sweetness that kids particularly love. They go very well with our Pasta Sauce as shown in the picture opposite (see page 42) and served with Mashed Potato (see page 182) or gluten-free pasta. It's very easy to increase the quantities to feed the whole family.

Mini PORK MEATBALLS

200g minced pork
½ small apple,
    finely grated
¼ small onion, very
    finely chopped
1 teaspoon fresh parsley
    leaves, finely chopped
Olive oil, for drizzling
Freshly ground black
    pepper

1 Preheat the oven to 200°C/180°C fan/400°F/Gas mark 6.

2 Combine all the ingredients really well in a bowl and with damp hands form into small equal-sized meatballs. If you don't wet your hands with a little water first, the meat will stick to your hands and will be harder to shape.

3 Heat a little oil in an ovenproof frying pan over a high heat. Fry the meatballs for a couple of minutes until they take on some colour. Transfer the pan to the oven for a further 8 minutes or until the meatballs are cooked through.

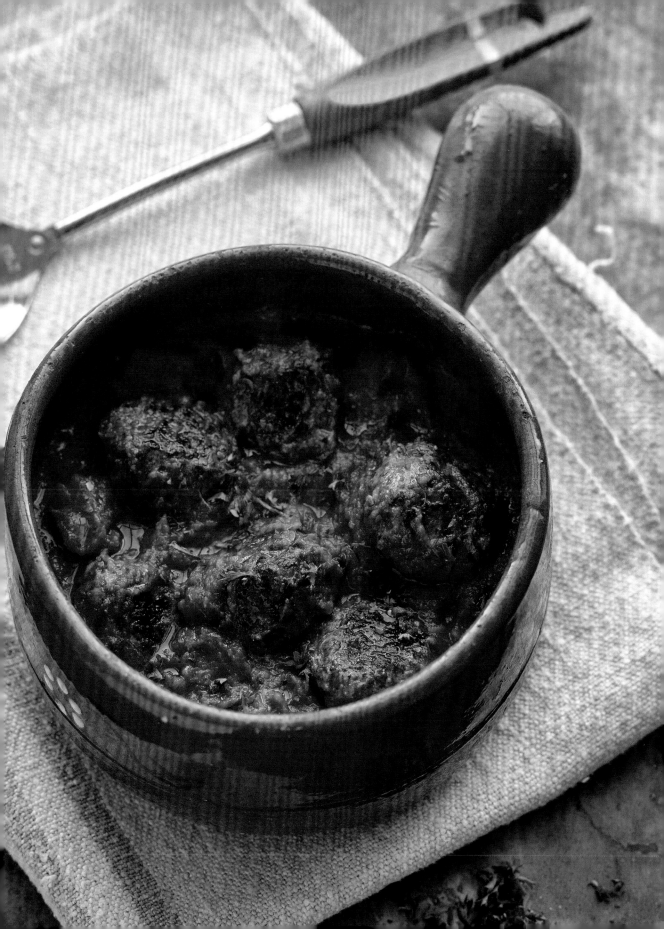

PREP: 5 MINUTES
COOK: 10 MINUTES

This is a really quick and easy recipe that not only works well for a supper dish, but can be used for a hearty breakfast too. Casper really likes this with pan-fried mashed potato and a good dollop of ketchup.

GAMMON *and Pineapple*

1 large gammon
   steak, cut in half
   (or 2 small ones)
2 rings of tinned
   pineapple, drained

1 Heat a little oil in a frying or griddle pan over a medium to high heat. Fry the gammon steaks for 4 minutes on each side. Check the gammon is cooked through.

2 Serve with cold pineapple rings on top.

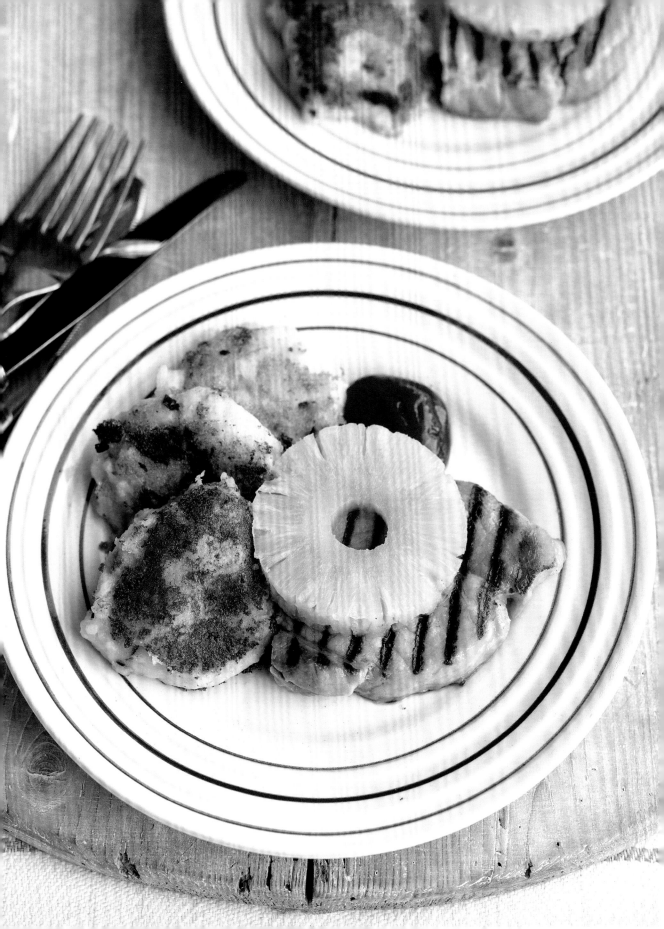

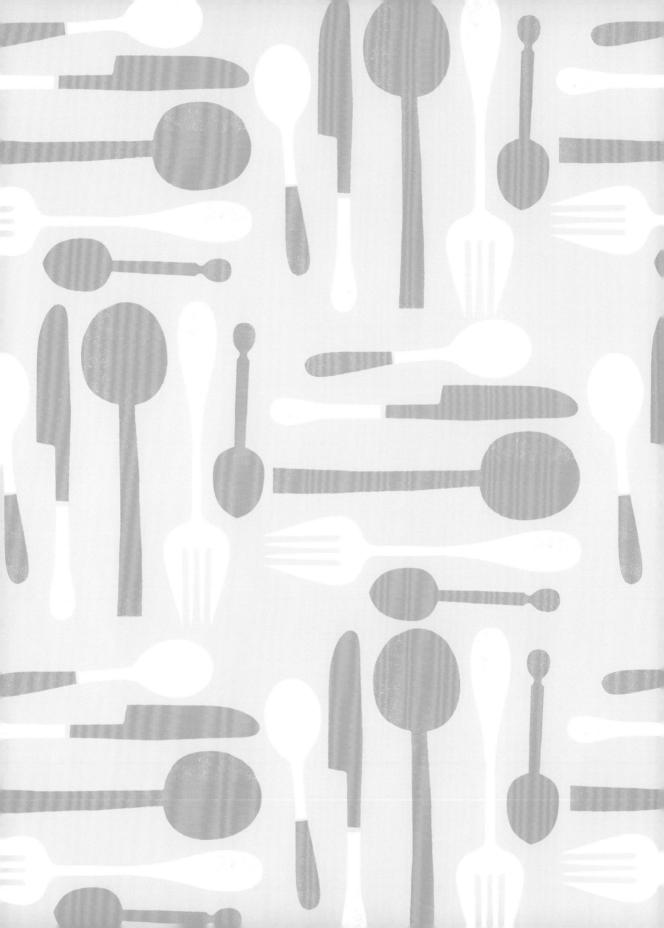

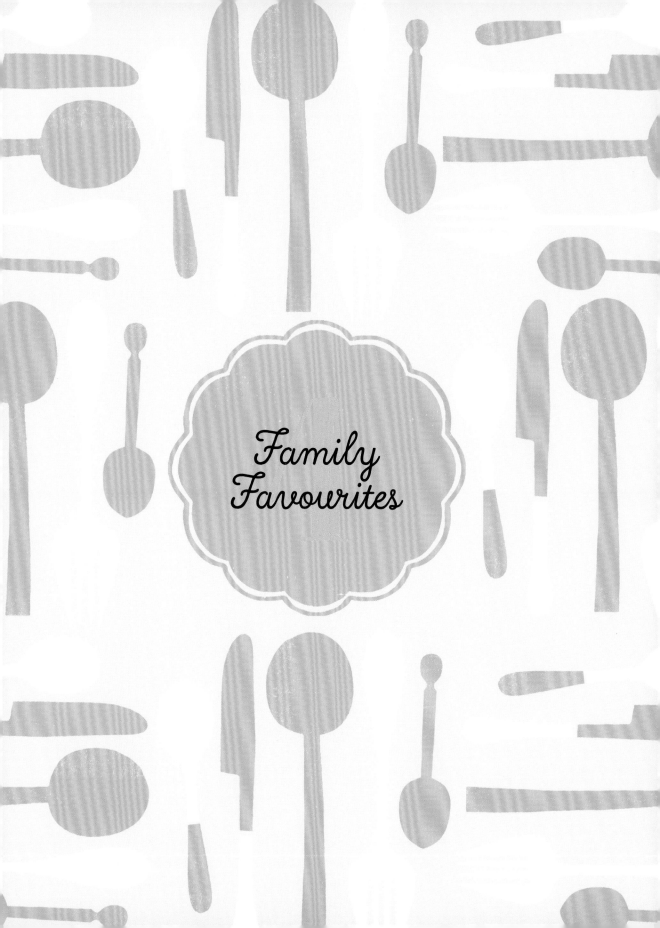

Family
Favourites

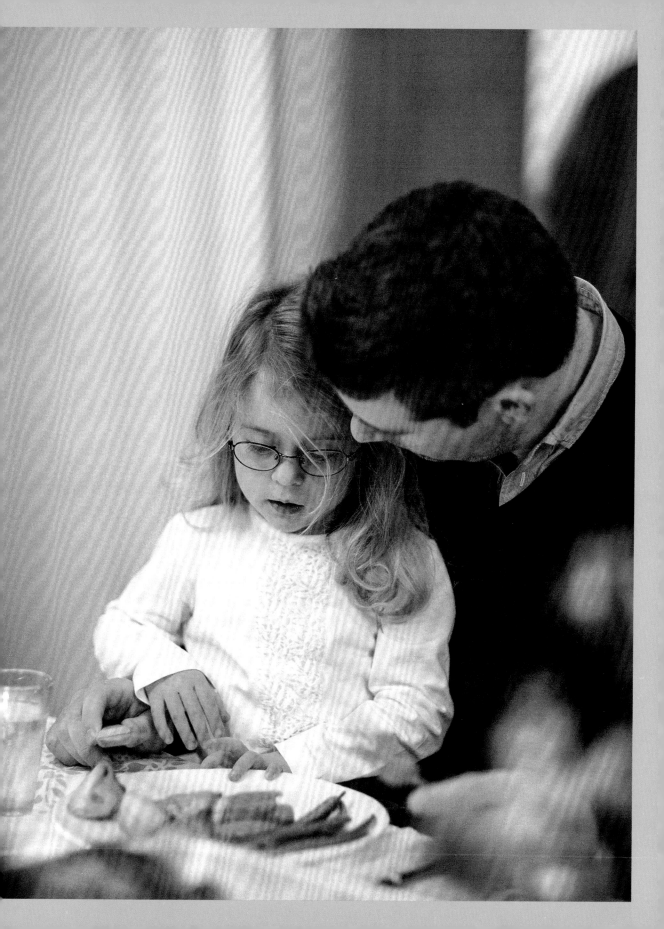

This is a really tasty, warming stew, which can also be blended to make a hearty soup. Ellie's sister is a vegetarian so we often cook this when she comes to stay with her family and it's always a big hit with everyone.

Lentil and Vegetable STEW

1 tablespoon olive oil
1 small red onion, sliced
1 small courgette, chopped
1 leek, chopped
1 large carrot, peeled and chopped
1 celery stick, chopped (optional)
6 cherry tomatoes
3 average-size new potatoes, roughly chopped
30g red split lentils (ones that do not require pre-soaking)
30g green lentils (ones that do not require pre-soaking)
½ 400g tin kidney beans, drained and rinsed
500ml fresh Vegetable Stock (see page 248) or ½ low-salt vegetable stock cube ❗ dissolved in 500ml boiling water
Freshly ground black pepper

1 Heat the oil in a pan. Fry the onion for a few minutes over a medium heat until softened.

2 Add all the other ingredients to the pan. If the stock does not cover the vegetables, then add extra water until everything in the pan is covered.

3 Cover with a lid and simmer for 35 minutes, stirring occasionally, checking that the lentils are tender before serving.

If you are not allergic

Add the optional celery. Serve with a tablespoon of crème fraîche on the side.

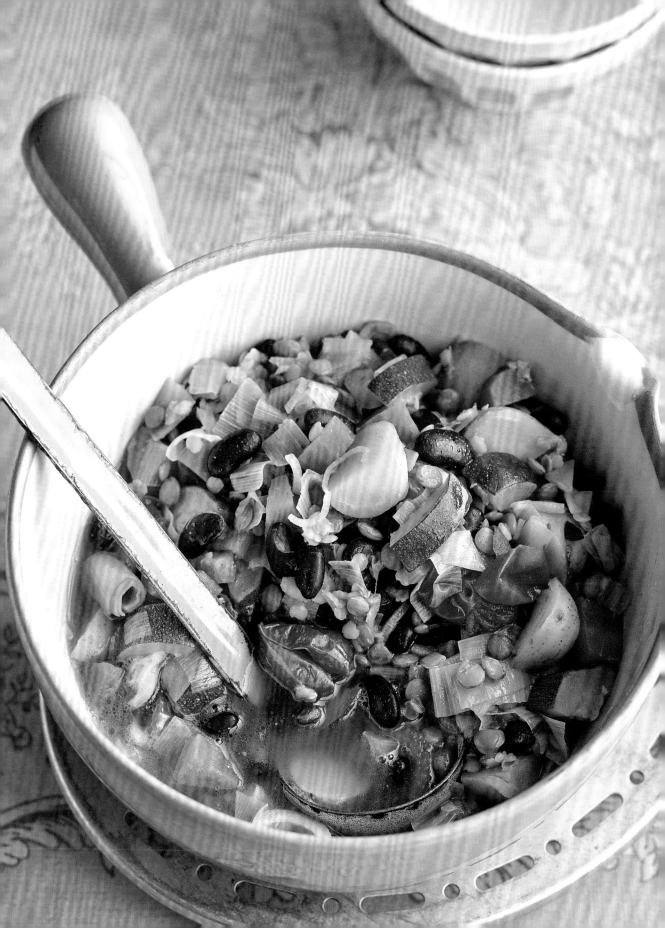

PREP: 10 MINUTES
COOK: 30 MINUTES

A popular vegetarian dish, stuffed peppers make a tasty and healthy meal. Use up any leftover vegetables you have to hand (spinach, mushrooms, broccoli and peas all work well) and if you want to make the meal more substantial you can stuff extra peppers with some cooked Chilli Con Carne (see page 54). If you prefer a more adult taste, add a sprinkle of dried chilli flakes when serving.

Vegetarian STUFFED PEPPERS

200g long-grain rice
3 red, green or yellow
    peppers, cut in half
    and deseeded
Large handful fine
    green beans, chopped
6 baby sweetcorn,
    chopped into rounds
1 courgette, chopped
    into small pieces
1 teaspoon olive oil
½ onion, finely chopped
2 garlic cloves, crushed
2 tomatoes, chopped

If you are not allergic
This is great with
a sprinkle of cheese
on top.

1 Preheat the oven to 220°C/200°C fan/425°F/Gas mark 7.

2 Boil the rice in a saucepan of water for 15 minutes or as per the instructions on your packet. Keep an eye on the timings and be ready to drain when cooked and set aside ready to use.

3 Meanwhile, in another pan of water, boil the peppers for 5 minutes. Use a slotted spoon to remove the peppers from the water and place them on a baking tray. Pop them into the oven for about 5–10 minutes while you prepare the stuffing.

4 Using the same pan of water used for the peppers, cook the beans, baby corn and courgette for a couple of minutes. Drain and set aside for a moment.

5 Using the same pan again now it is empty, heat the oil and lightly fry the onion for a few minutes until softened. Add the garlic and cook for a further minute. Remove from the heat and then add the vegetables you have just cooked and drained.

6 The rice should be cooked by now, so add this to the pan along with the tomatoes and stir well.

7 Remove the peppers from the oven and fill with the rice mixture, drizzle with a little olive oil and return to the oven for a further 5 minutes. If you have extra rice then simply serve on the side.

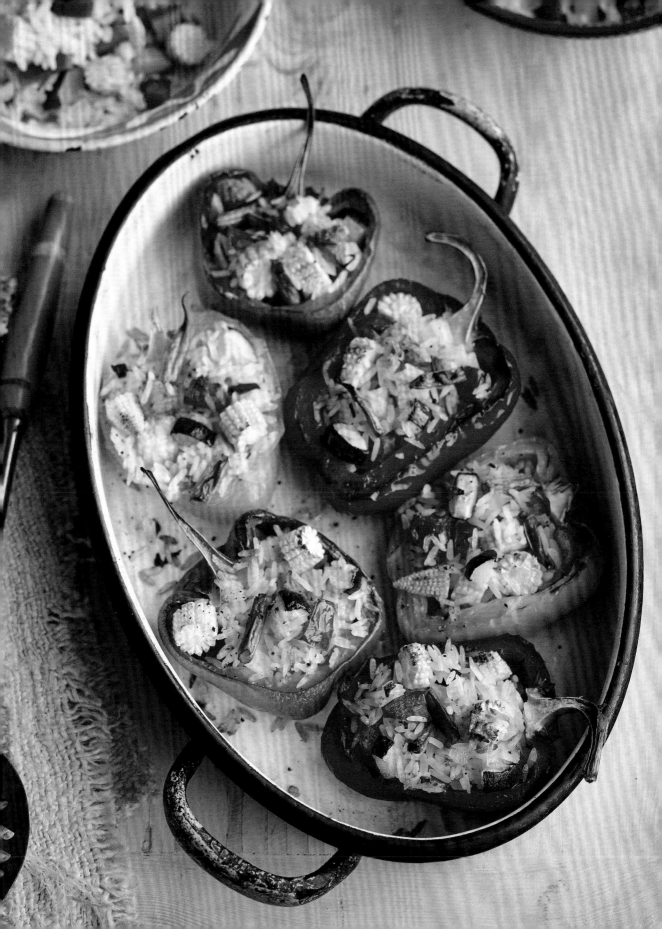

SERVES A FAMILY OF 4

PREP: 5 MINUTES
COOK: 15 MINUTES

This curry has lovely Thai flavours and the tomatoes work brilliantly with fish, but you could easily omit the fish to make a vegetarian curry. The mild flavours suit kids but simply add more of our Homemade Southeast Asian Blend (see page 251) if you prefer a stronger taste, and a little chilli if you want some heat. Coley, salmon, tilapia or pollock all work very well in this recipe. This curry is particularly nice for those who can't have dairy as it has a lovely creaminess from the coconut milk.

Mild FISH CURRY

Olive oil, for drizzling
4 tablespoons Homemade Southeast Asian Blend (see page 251)
400g tin coconut milk
400g tin chopped tomatoes
4 x 100g portions of skinless firm fish fillets of your choice, chopped into chunks
16 baby sweetcorn, cut into pieces
2 handfuls fine green beans, chopped into pieces
2 bulbs pak choi, sliced lengthways
2 handfuls fresh coriander, chopped

1 Heat a little oil in a pan over a medium to high heat. Gently fry the Southeast Asian Blend in the pan for a moment, allowing the shallots to soften.

2 Add the coconut milk, coconut cream, if using, and tomatoes to the pan. Bring to a gentle simmer and allow to cook for 5 minutes.

3 Add the fish and vegetables and then cook gently for a further 5 minutes or until the fish is cooked and the vegetables are tender.

4 Garnish with coriander before serving.

VARIATION
Increase the quantity of vegetables or add different vegetables such as peas or courgettes or whatever your children particularly like to turn this into a vegetarian curry, omitting the fish at step 3.

Optional Extras
You can also add a small tin or carton of coconut cream if your child needs feeding up.

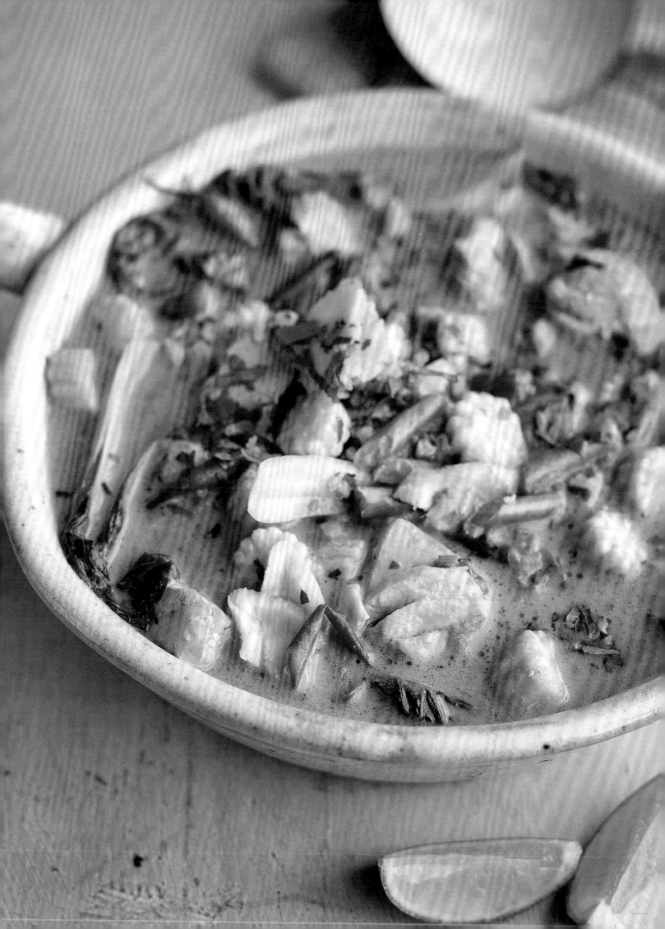

This is a really easy supper dish with a subtle lemon flavour. It makes a nice alternative to a traditional Sunday roast and is delicious served simply with the pan juices, Roast Potatoes (see page 178) and lots of vegetables. Buying a whole chicken is a lot more economical than buying chicken pieces and the leftover bones are great for making your own stock (see page 250). The Vietnamese Rice Noodle Soup (see page 81) and Chicken and Mango Salad (see page 84) are both tasty ways of using up any leftover pieces of chicken.

SERVES
A FAMILY OF
4

with some leftovers

PREP: 5 MINUTES
COOK: 1 HOUR

Lemon ROAST CHICKEN

1.5kg whole chicken
2 lemons, cut into
 quarters
Olive oil, for drizzling
Handful fresh parsley,
 chopped
125ml water
Freshly ground black
 pepper

1 Preheat the oven to 220°C/200°C fan/425°F/Gas mark 7.

2 Place the chicken in a roasting tin. Open the cavity of the chicken and push in the lemon quarters.

3 Drizzle some olive oil over the skin and grind over some freshly ground black pepper. Scatter the parsley on top.

4 Add the water to the bottom of the pan – this will help keep the chicken moist and form a good base for a sauce.

5 Roast according to the exact weight of the chicken – a 1.5kg chicken will cook in about 1 hour. As a rule of thumb, chickens should be cooked for 40 minutes per kilo.

6 When the chicken is cooked transfer it to a carving board to rest for a few minutes. Always check that the chicken is cooked by cutting in at the thigh – if the juices are at all pink or bloody the chicken is not cooked. Only serve when the juices run clear.

7 Skim off any excess fat from the pan juices ready to be served as a simple, light gravy. If preferred, the pan juices can be thickened. Simply mix a teaspoon of cornflour with a tablespoon of cold water in a small bowl and then add to the pan juices and bring to a simmer.

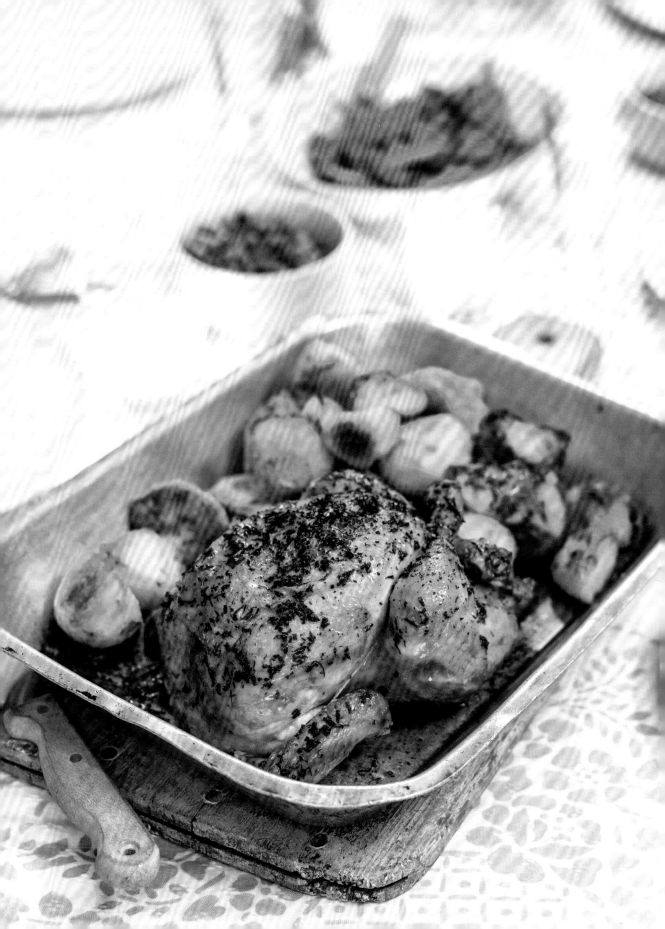

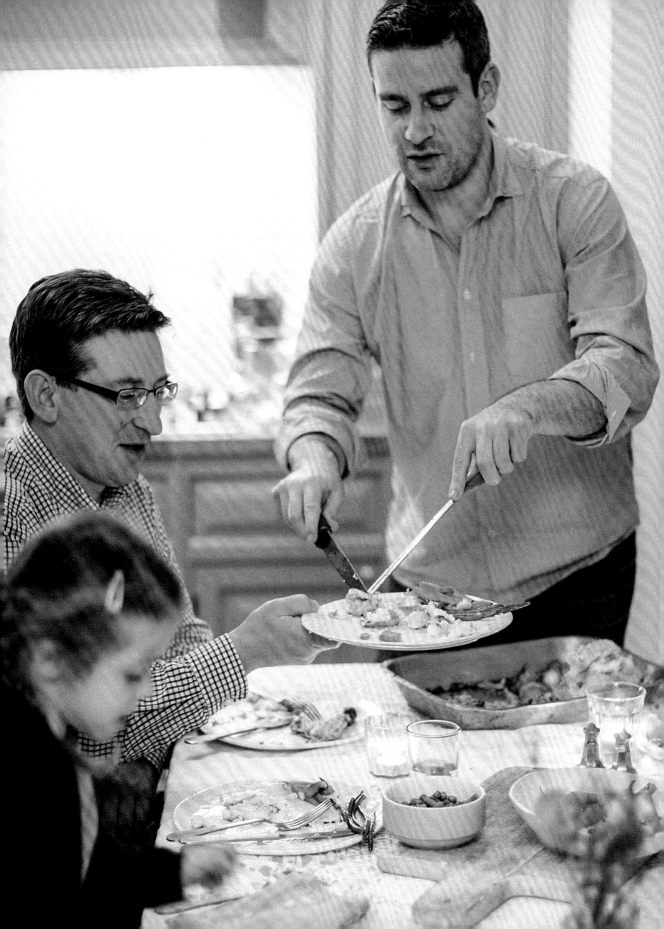

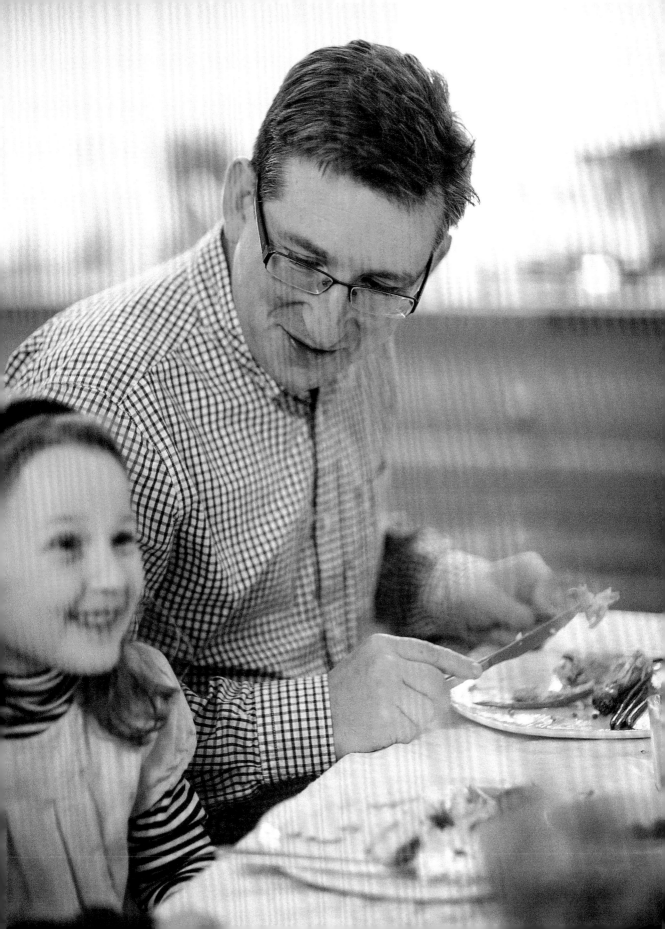

PREP: 5 MINUTES
COOK: 30 MINUTES

Paella normally contains seafood but our version is made with tender pieces of chicken and vegetables and is really tasty. This is a similar concept to risotto in that the whole meal is cooked in one pan but it's a bit easier as paella rice doesn't need constant stirring. This is a great all-in-one supper dish for any time of the year.

Spanish CHICKEN PAELLA

1 tablespoon olive oil

4 boneless, skinless chicken thighs

2 tablespoons chopped cooking chorizo (!) (optional)

1 red pepper, deseeded and chopped

½ onion, chopped

2 garlic cloves, crushed

200g paella rice

A few strands of saffron or 1 teaspoon turmeric (see note below)

850ml fresh Chicken Stock (see page 250) or ½ low-salt chicken stock cube (!) dissolved in 850ml boiling water

1 small courgette, cut into quarters and then into small slices

Handful fine green beans, chopped

3 broccoli florets, broken into small pieces

1 Heat the oil in a large frying pan over a medium-high heat and fry the chicken pieces and chorizo, if using, for about 5 minutes, allowing them to take on a little colour.

2 Add the pepper and onion and allow to soften for a minute or two.

3 Add the garlic, rice and saffron (or turmeric) and stir for a couple of minutes. Keep stirring to make sure the rice doesn't stick to the bottom of your pan and all the ingredients combine well.

4 Pour over the stock, bring to the boil and then turn down and gently simmer for 10 minutes.

5 Add the courgette, beans and broccoli and then gently simmer for a further 10 minutes.

6 Stir once just to check that the rice has not stuck to the bottom of the pan.

If you are not allergic
Stir in a handful of cooked prawns at the end of cooking.

Note
The saffron gives the lovely yellow colour to the rice but it is very expensive so turmeric makes a great everyday alternative.

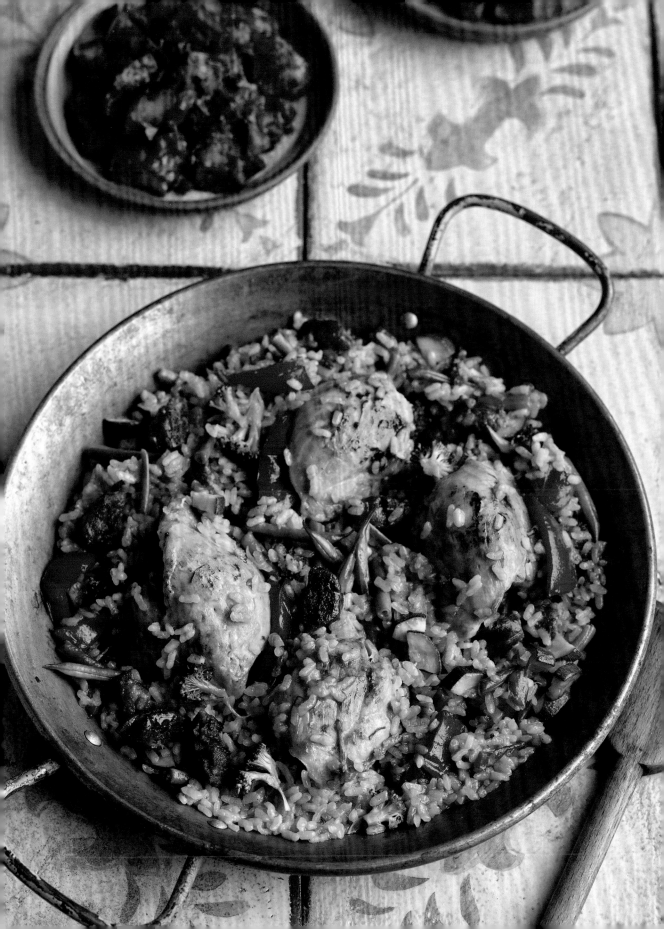

This is a mild dish, not hot in the slightest – it just contains lovely aromatic spices and creamy coconut milk and is a gentle way to introduce children to Indian flavours. Often you will find ready-made korma sauces or pastes that are made with nuts, usually almonds. This recipe has no nuts and uses spices that you would typically have in your larder. When we cook for lots of kids this is a big hit, especially when served with vegetables, Coconut Rice (see page 194), poppadoms, chutneys and dips.

Ever-so-Mild
CHICKEN KORMA

2 teaspoons olive oil

1 onion, peeled and quartered

2 teaspoons ground coriander

1 teaspoon ground turmeric

½ teaspoon ground ginger

Small pinch salt (optional)

Good pinch sugar

1 teaspoon coriander seeds

3 large skinless chicken breasts, cut into chunks

400ml tin coconut milk

8 cardamom pods

Handful fresh coriander, chopped

Flaked coconut, to garnish (optional)

1 Put the oil, onion, ground coriander, turmeric, ginger, salt (if using) and sugar in a blender and blitz to a smooth paste.

2 Heat the paste and the coriander seeds in a pan over a medium heat and stir for a minute. Add the chicken, stir so that it is coated with the paste and keep stirring for a further minute.

3 Add the coconut milk and cardamom pods, cover and simmer for about 8 minutes, making sure the chicken is cooked through before serving.

4 Remove the cardamom pods and garnish with a little chopped coriander and flaked coconut.

VARIATION

If you want to make a Lamb Korma, use an ovenproof casserole and follow the recipe as above, replacing the chicken with 200g diced lamb neck and add 250ml water with the coconut milk. Bring to a simmer and pop into a preheated oven at 180°C/160°C fan/350°F/Gas mark 4 and cook for about 1–1½ hours. Check that the lamb is nice and tender before serving.

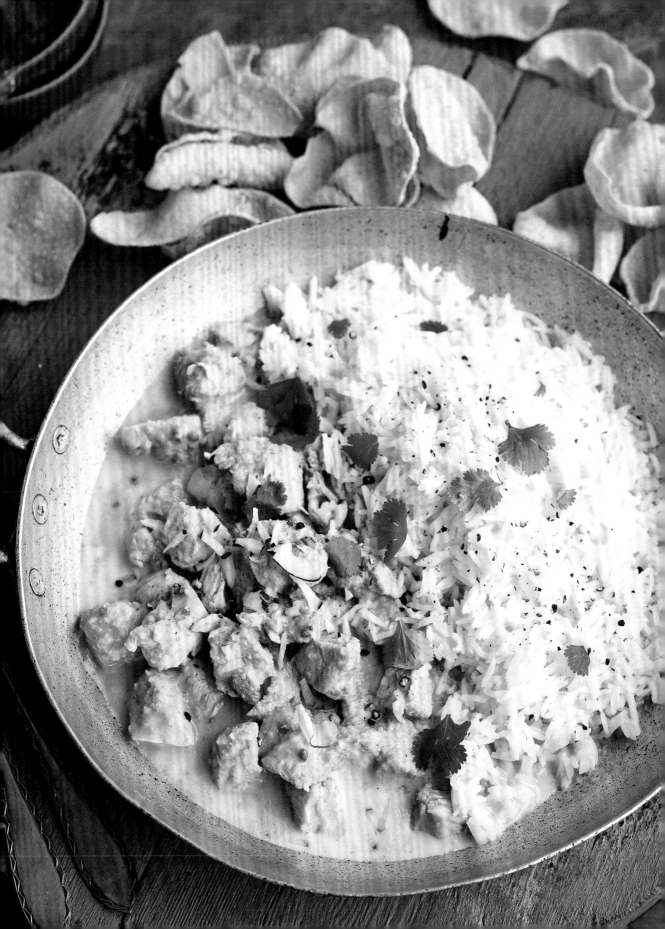

This is a fabulous retro dish that was very popular in the Seventies. You might not think to give your kids duck but ours love this meal and they especially like the combination of duck with fresh tangy orange. It goes well with wild rice and green vegetables such as broccoli and mange tout. If you have more time, it is also delicious with our Boulangère Potatoes (see page 174) and if you want to continue the Seventies theme you can serve our Chocolate Fondue (see page 230) with strawberries for dessert!

SERVES A FAMILY OF 4

PREP: 5 MINUTES
COOK: 25 MINUTES

Retro
DUCK À L'ORANGE

3 duck breasts,
    with skin left on
1 orange, cut into
    quarters
2 shallots, finely chopped
2 carrots, peeled
    and chopped
1 bay leaf
Olive oil, for drizzling
200ml orange juice

1 Preheat the oven to 220°C/200°C fan/425°F/Gas mark 7.

2 Prick the skin of the duck breasts with a fork or score with a sharp knife (making sure you don't cut through to the flesh) – this will help some of the fat come out of the skin and make it nice and crispy.

3 Sear the duck breasts, skin side down, in a frying pan over a high heat until the skin looks golden – you will not need any oil for this as there is plenty of fat in the skin.

4 Arrange the seared duck breasts, skin side up, in a roasting tin and tuck the orange pieces, shallots, carrots and bay leaf around them. Drizzle with a little oil.

5 Roast in the oven until the duck is just cooked through to your liking. This should take about 15 minutes for the meat to be medium and 18 minutes for the meat to be well done.

6 Remove the duck from the pan to rest for a moment while you make the sauce. Add the orange juice to the roasting tin and give it a good stir, then strain into a small saucepan and place over a high heat to reduce down a little. Skim off any excess fat.

7 Slice the duck breasts and pour the sauce over the top to serve.

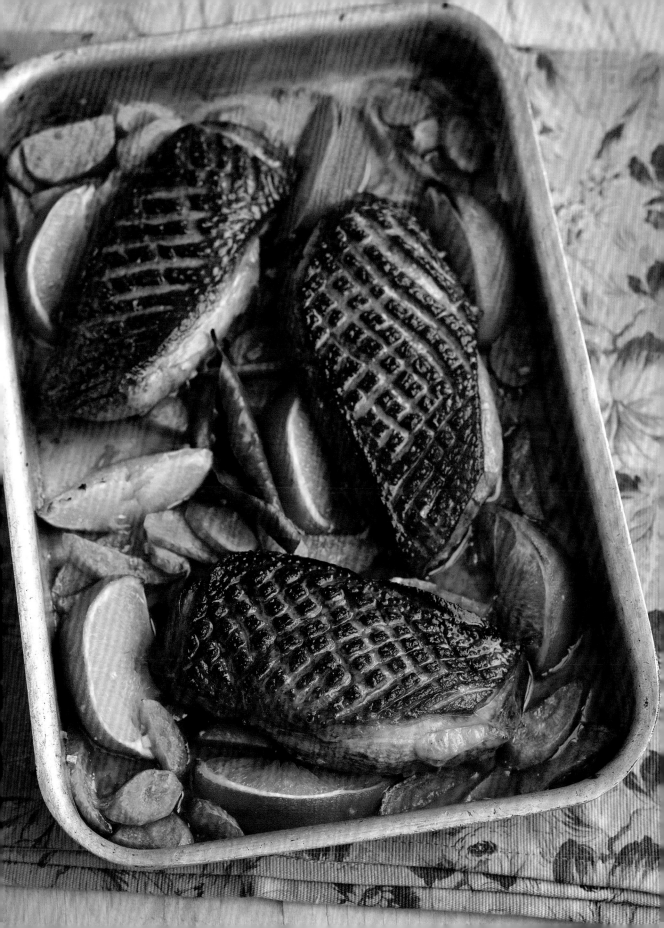

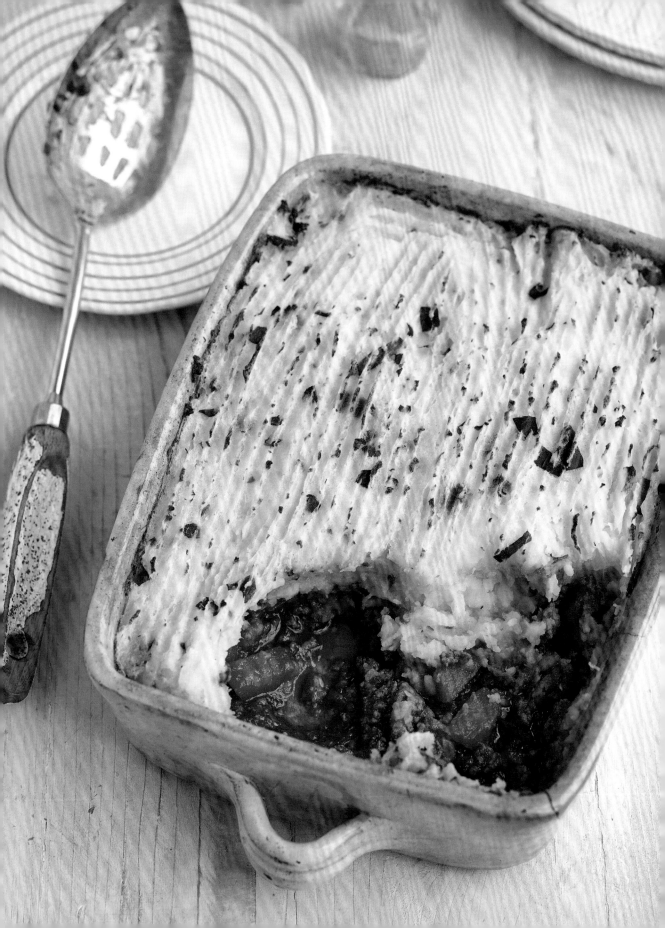

This is a traditional supper dish and a favourite with most families. You can also use beef instead of lamb to make a cottage pie if you prefer. Shepherd's pie is normally topped with mashed potato but if you want to try a different version just slice up some peeled potatoes and layer them on top before popping in the oven; it makes a lovely crunchy alternative. It is delicious either way and is best served with garden peas or broccoli and tomato ketchup.

SERVES
A FAMILY OF
4

PREP: 15 MINUTES
COOK: 2 HOURS

SHEPHERD'S PIE

2 tablespoons olive oil
500g lamb mince
1 onion, chopped
400g tin chopped
    tomatoes
200ml fresh Vegetable
    Stock (see page 248)
    or ½ low-salt vegetable
    stock cube ❗
    dissolved in 200ml
    boiling water
3 carrots, peeled, halved
    and chopped
Mashed Potato (see page
    182), for the topping

1 Preheat the oven to 180°C/160°C fan/350°F/Gas mark 4.

2 Heat the oil in a large heavy-based, ovenproof pan over a medium to high heat and add the lamb mince, bit by bit, allowing it to get some colour, but being careful not to let it burn. It is best not to move the mince about too much.

3 Add the onion and cook for a few minutes, allowing it to soften. Add the tomatoes, stock and carrots and bring to a simmer.

4 Put a lid on the pan and pop it into the oven for 1½ hours, giving it a quick stir every 30 minutes or so. If needed, add extra water if the mixture is starting to look a little dry. Don't skimp on the cooking time – this dish really needs it to allow the meat to become very tender and to create a thick sauce around the meat.

5 Remove from the oven and skim off any excess fat with a spoon (don't be alarmed if there is a lot of fat on the surface as lamb can be quite a fatty meat).

6 Tip the meat into an ovenproof serving dish and top with the mashed potato. Run a fork over the mash to make lines across the top and pop the dish in the oven for 10 more minutes to crisp up.

This is a big favourite in both our households served with a gluten-free bun, oven chips with free-from mayonnaise and a nice green salad. It is so easy and quick to make your own burgers; please don't be put off by the capers, they just add a depth of flavour rather than a strong taste. The burgers are easy to make a day in advance, just cover and refrigerate them or you can freeze them while raw, making sure that the individual burgers are wrapped in greaseproof paper so they are easy to separate when defrosted. Don't be tempted to buy low-fat content beef mince as you need the fat to keep the burger moist and sticking together.

MAKES 8 BURGERS

PREP: 10 MINUTES
COOK: 8 MINUTES

Homemade BEEF BURGERS

500g beef mince
½ small onion, very finely chopped
1½ tablespoons capers, drained, rinsed and chopped
1 teaspoon grated zest from an unwaxed lemon
1 small garlic clove, crushed
Small handful fresh parsley, chopped
Pinch salt (optional)
Freshly ground black pepper

1 Preheat the oven to 220°C/200°C fan/425°F/Gas mark 7.

2 Mix all the ingredients really well in a bowl and form into burgers with your hands (each burger should be about 70g). Wet your hands slightly to stop the meat sticking to them.

3 Heat a little oil in an ovenproof frying pan and cook the burgers over a medium to high heat until they have some colour on the outside. Pop the pan in the oven for about 6–8 minutes until the meat is cooked through. Be careful not to overcook otherwise the burgers can become a bit dry.

....

Optional Extras
These burgers may be a little plain for grown-ups but you can easily add ½ teaspoon ground cumin and a good pinch of cayenne pepper to half of the mixture if preferred – just remember which ones are which when serving!

If you are not allergic
Serve with a sesame seed bun, mayo and a slice of cheese.

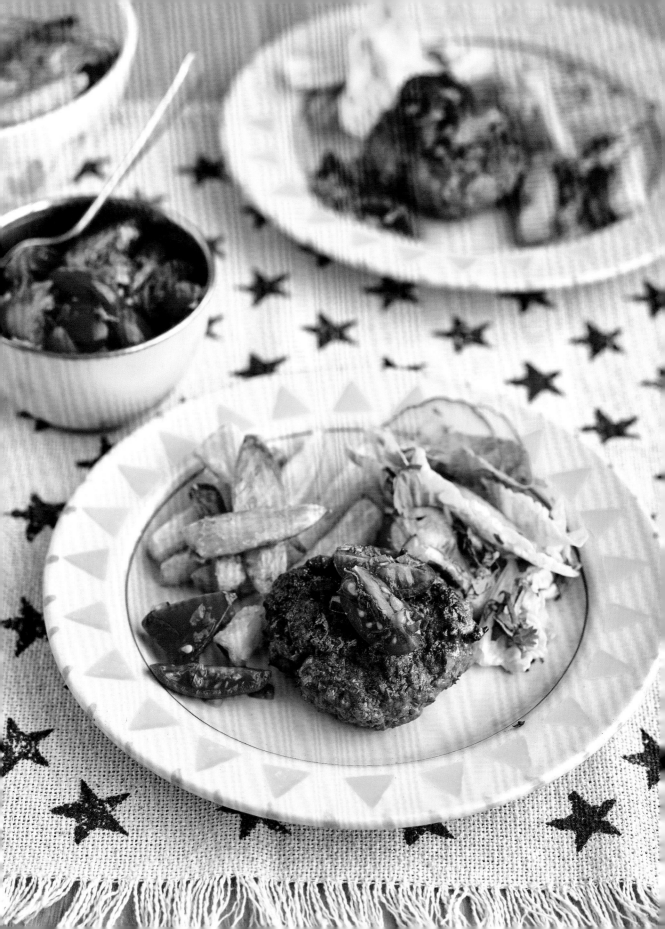

These lamb kebabs include a variety of interesting flavours, which are great to introduce your kids to. Don't be tempted to buy low-fat content lamb mince (the fat ensures a moist, lovely kebab and a lot of the fat will will be rendered down during the cooking process anyway). These are great served with our sesame-free Hummus (see page 132) and Cucumber Salsa (see page 137). Both our families like these kebabs served with our Pilau Rice with Fruit (see page 196), gluten-free pitta breads or Potato Wedges (see page 184). The kebabs can be prepared a day in advance. You can also freeze the skewers while still raw, but remember to defrost fully before grilling.

MAKES 12 KEBABS

PREP: 10 MINUTES
COOK: 10 MINUTES

Greek LAMB KEBABS

12 bamboo or metal kebab sticks (if you are using bamboo skewers soak in water for 30 minutes beforehand)
1 shallot, finely chopped
500g lamb mince
2 garlic cloves, crushed
2 teaspoons ground coriander
1 tablespoon ground cumin
2 teaspoons lemon juice
1 tablespoon chopped fresh coriander leaves

1 Put all the ingredients in a bowl and mix together really well with your hands. Or if you prefer just blitz everything quickly in a mixer.

2 Use your hands to press about 45g of meat onto each kebab skewer and mould the mixture around it. At this point you can cover with clingfilm and pop into the fridge until you're ready to cook.

3 Preheat the grill to a medium to high heat. Cook the kebabs under the hot grill for about 7–8 minutes until cooked and lightly browned, turning as necessary to ensure even cooking. Alternatively, you could cook the kebabs in an oven preheated to 220°C/200°C fan/425°F/ Gas mark 7 for a similar amount of time.

Optional Extras
Feel free to add more of the spice and, if your family can tolerate a little heat, add a teaspoon of cayenne pepper for a more grown-up kebab.

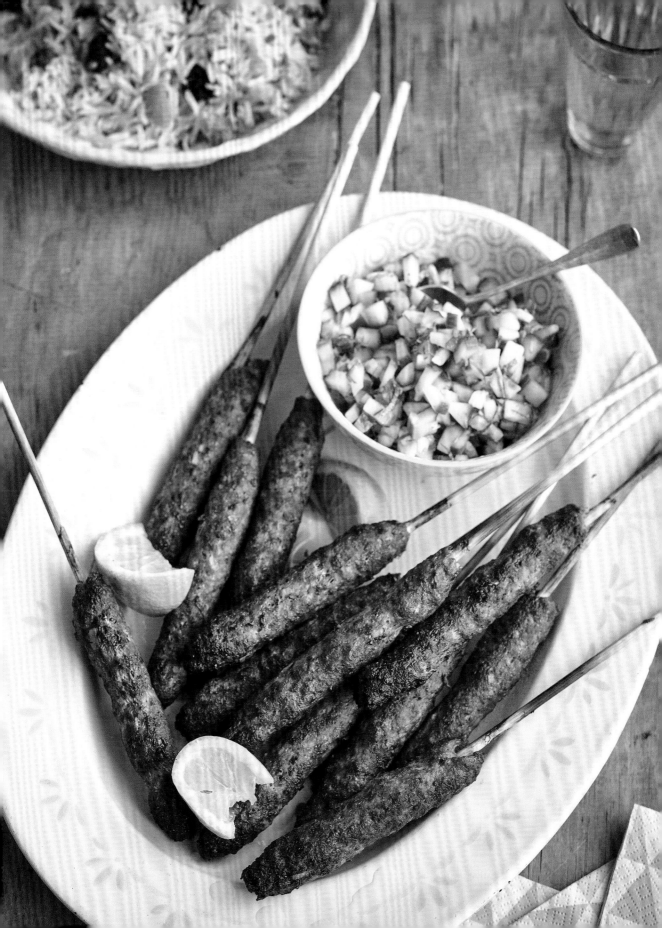

PREP: 15 MINUTES
COOK: 40 MINUTES

This is really lovely for an easy Sunday lunch and delicious with the apple sauce and with our gravy too (see page 249). The pork fillet is very tender so great for young kids and a big hit with both of our families. The apple sauce freezes well so you can make a large batch and freeze in portions.

PORK FILLET
with Apple Sauce

500g pork fillet
6 streaky bacon rashers
Handful fresh sage leaves
Handful fresh parsley
   leaves, chopped
¼ small onion, finely
   chopped
1 large garlic clove,
   crushed
Freshly ground black
   pepper
Oil, for drizzling

Apple sauce
1 large cooking apple,
   peeled and core
   removed (about 200g)
1 strip of unwaxed
   lemon peel
1 teaspoon lemon juice
1 teaspoon brown sugar
   (adjust according
   to your own taste)
1 teaspoon water

1 Preheat the oven to 220°C/200°C fan/425°F/Gas mark 7.

2 Trim any excess fat or sinew from the pork fillet. Cover a chopping board with some food-safe clingfilm and then lay out the bacon in strips in a line on top.

3 Sprinkle the bacon with the sage leaves, parsley, onion, garlic and a little pepper to taste.

4 Place the pork fillet on top of the bacon at the front edge of the board and then with the help of the clingfilm roll it up, wrapping the bacon around the pork fillet as tightly as you can.

5 Wrap the whole thing in clingfilm, and if preparing in advance, pop it in the fridge until you are ready to roast it.

6 Remove the clingfilm and place the pork in a roasting tin. Drizzle with a little oil and pop it in the oven for about 30 minutes until the meat is cooked through.

7 Meanwhile, make the apple sauce. Chop the apple into large chunks and put in a pan with the lemon peel, lemon juice, sugar and water. Cover with a lid and cook over a low heat, stirring occasionally, for about 20 minutes until the apple has broken down into a soft sauce. Remove the lemon peel and leave the sauce to cool before serving.

8 When the pork has cooked, leave it to rest for at least 5 minutes before slicing and serving with apple sauce.

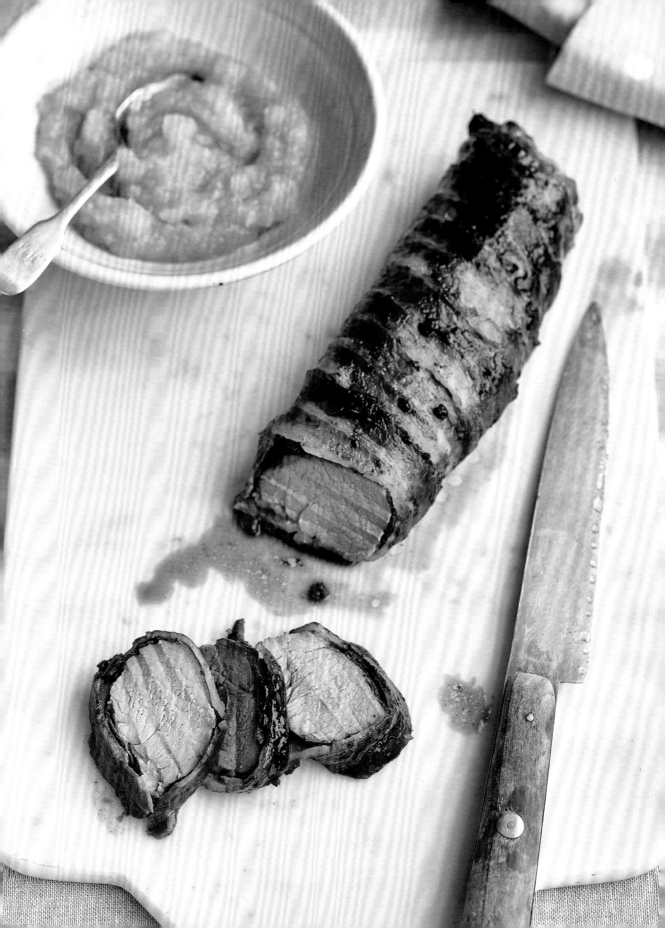

There's nothing nicer than sitting down together to eat as a family and really enjoying a hearty meal. Although these recipes take slightly longer to prepare compared with our super-quick suppers, they are worth it as a lot of the extra time is taken up while the dish is in the oven. So although the overall cooking time is longer, you won't be slaving away for hours. We tend to eat a lot of these meals as a family at the weekend.

We feel it is very important to share the same meal, allergy or no allergy. Often during the week the kids will have tea after school separately so it is really nice to have family time at the kitchen table where everyone is included. These recipes are great for both adults and kids and also work very well if you're having other families over for lunch.

We also eat a lot of traditional roasts, which are generally a good option for allergy sufferers if you make your own gravy (see page 249) and ensure you don't use butter to baste a chicken. Our children love to have a roast at the weekend and we have included a couple of nice recipes to give you a more interesting twist on roast chicken and roast pork.

Most of these recipes are designed with a family of four in mind but we appreciate you may be cooking for more or fewer people and children's portion sizes vary depending on their age, so the amounts can easily be adapted to suit you.

SERVES A FAMILY OF 4

PREP: 10 MINUTES
COOK: 15 MINUTES

This is a great classic of Chinese cuisine and a favourite on takeaway menus, but if you have allergies it can often be hard to find a suitable restaurant or takeaway that is safe for your set of allergies. Well, fear not – this is so simple and even better than many takeaway dishes we have tried, so nobody needs to miss out. This is great served with boiled long-grain rice and baby sweetcorn.

Chinese-Style SWEET AND SOUR PORK

1 teaspoon cornflour

2 tablespoons water

2 tablespoons granulated sugar

2 tablespoons orange juice, from a carton

1 teaspoon tomato purée

2 teaspoons white wine vinegar

⅛ teaspoon salt (optional)

1 teaspoon olive oil

½ small onion, sliced

1 red pepper, deseeded and chopped into chunks

500g pork fillet, trimmed of any sinews and sliced

½ teaspoon Chinese five-spice (see Note below)

140g tin pineapple in juice, chopped into chunks

50g tinned bamboo shoots (optional)

1 Mix together the cornflour and water in a small bowl. Add the sugar, orange juice, tomato purée, white wine vinegar and salt (if using). Mix together and then set aside.

2 Heat the oil in a frying pan over a medium to high heat and gently fry the onion and red pepper for a few minutes until they start to soften.

3 Add the pork slices and then cook for couple of minutes on each side until lightly browned and just cooked through.

4 Stir in the Chinese five-spice and cook for a further minute.

5 Add the cornflour mixture and the pineapple chunks and bamboo shoots, if using. Stir through and leave to simmer for a few moments. The sauce will start to bubble and thicken quite quickly. If you prefer a runnier sauce, just add a little water or juice from the pineapple tin before serving.

Note
Some Chinese five-spice seasoning packets have a whole range of added ingredients such as salt and sugar as well as allergens. Make sure yours contains just cinnamon, fennel, star anise, ginger and cloves.

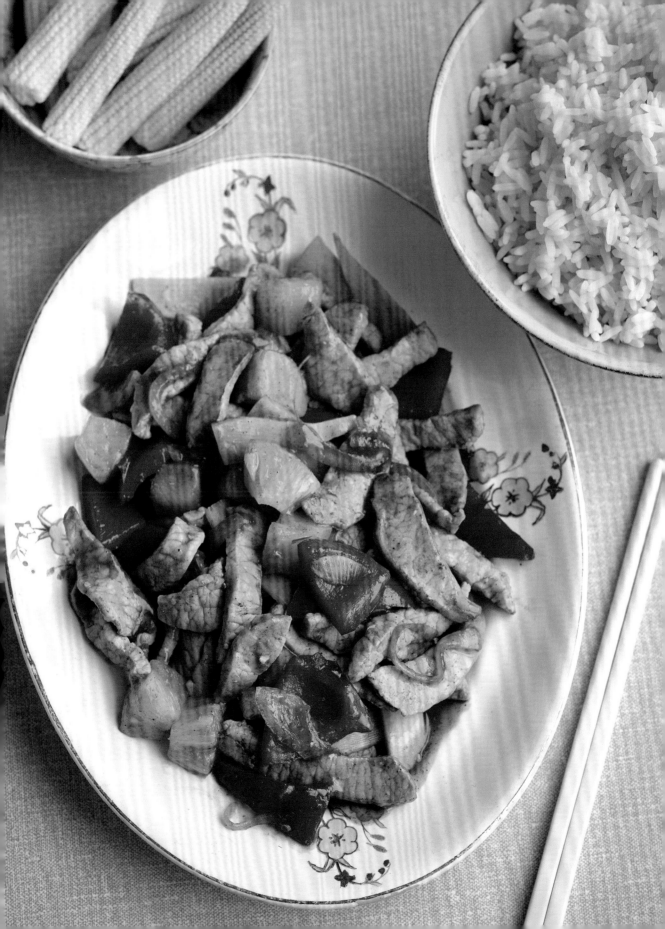

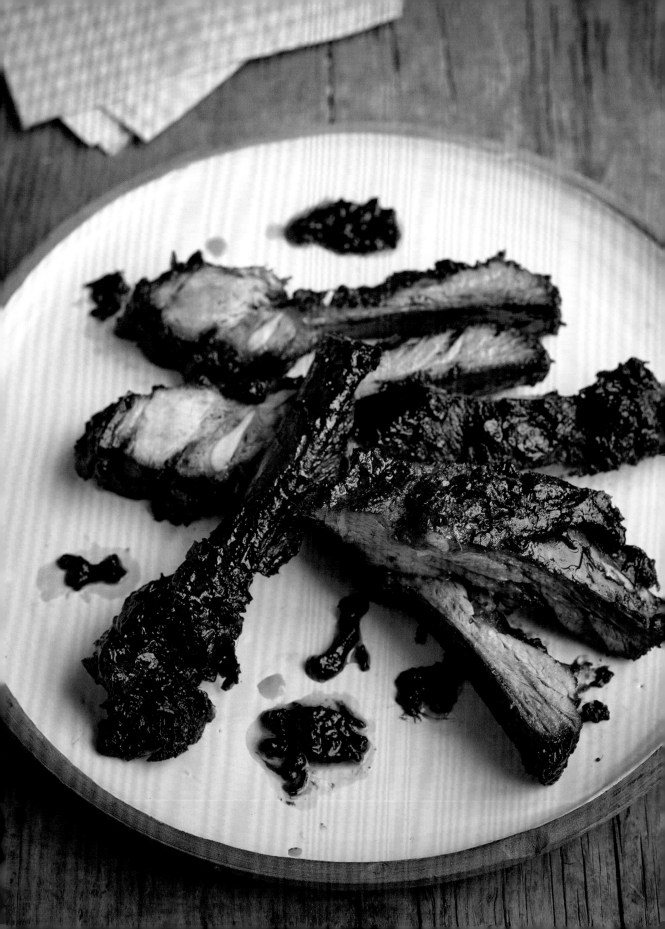

Our kids love sticky ribs, partly because they can eat with their fingers and get stuck in. Blackstrap molasses, which is relatively high in calcium, can replace the treacle and is a good addition to your child's diet if they can't have dairy.

Sticky SPARE RIBS

1 teaspoon olive oil

2 tablespoons tomato ketchup (low-salt and sugar ketchup is best)

1½ tablespoons finely chopped or grated fresh ginger

2 garlic cloves, crushed

1 small onion, finely chopped

3 tablespoons treacle or blackstrap molasses

2 tablespoons runny honey

1 tablespoon soft dark brown sugar

1 tablespoon white wine vinegar

¼ teaspoon Chinese five-spice (!) (see Note on page 122)

700g pork spare ribs

Freshly ground black pepper

1 Mix all the ingredients, except the spare ribs, in a bowl. Pour this marinade over the ribs in a suitable container and pop in the fridge to marinate for a few hours or overnight.

2 Preheat the oven to 200°C/180°C fan/400°F/Gas mark 6.

3 Place the marinated ribs on a baking tray so they fit snugly and pour over any remaining sauce left in the container.

4 Cook in the oven until the ribs are cooked through, checking every 10 minutes or so to give the tray a little shake and to keep the marinade moving about.

5 If you buy your ribs from a supermarket there will be cooking times on the packet, or ask your butcher. As a rule of thumb, cook ribs for 30 minutes per 500g plus an extra 20 minutes. If using the barbecue, we recommend cooking the ribs first in the oven and then finishing off on the barbecue.

6 Leave to cool a little before serving as the sticky sauce is very hot when it comes straight out of the oven.

VARIATION

This sticky marinade works equally well with chicken. Simply replace the spare ribs with 6 chicken drumsticks and cook for 25 minutes.

PREP: 5 MINUTES
COOK: 1 HOUR
20 MINUTES

This is a much-loved family supper dish and great in the colder months. Our version is not too rich so great for younger palates but still very tasty. Casper particularly likes this with Mashed Potato (see page 182) or Jacket Potatoes (see page 192) and plenty of vegetables such as sweetcorn and cauliflower.

Sausage and Bean
CASSEROLE

1 teaspoon olive oil
8 good-quality
   sausages
1 large red onion,
   halved and sliced
2 bacon rashers, chopped
2 large garlic cloves,
   crushed
125ml water
400g tin chopped
   tomatoes
400g tin haricot beans,
   drained and rinsed
   (kidney beans also
   work well if you happen
   to have a tin)
A few sprigs of fresh thyme
1 bay leaf
Freshly ground black
   pepper

1 Preheat the oven to 200°C/180°C fan/400°F/Gas mark 6.

2 Heat the oil in an ovenproof casserole and fry the sausages over a medium to high heat until they take on a little colour.

3 Add the onion and bacon and cook for a further few minutes, then add the garlic.

4 Pour the water into the pan and bring to a simmer. Add the tomatoes, haricot beans, thyme and bay leaf, cover with a lid and place in the oven for 1 hour.

5 Remove the lid for the last 5 minutes of cooking to reduce the sauce a little and allow the sausages sitting at the top to brown a little.

6 Skim off any excess fat from the top, remove the bay leaf and season to taste before serving.

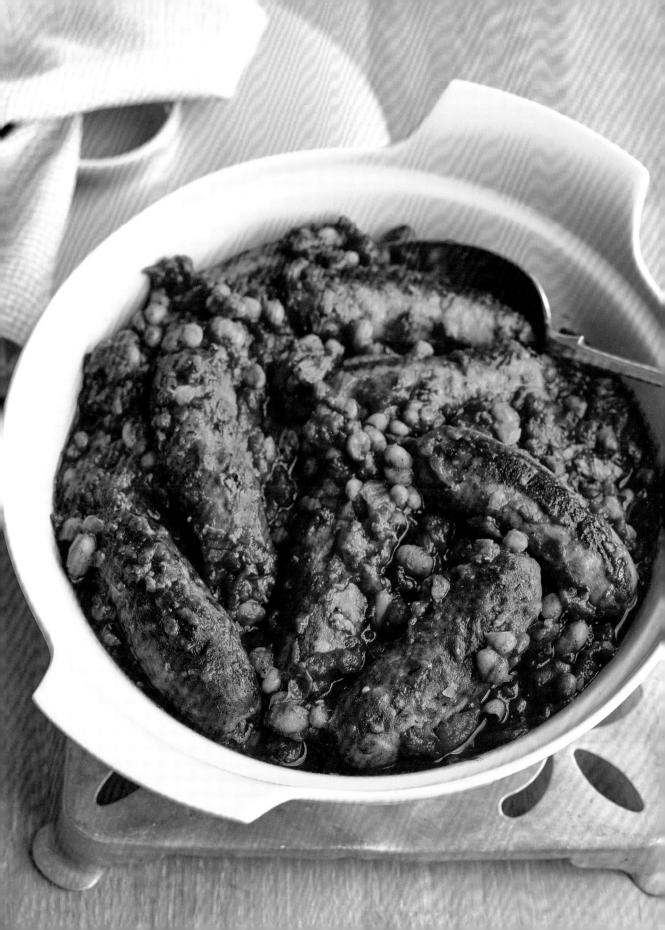

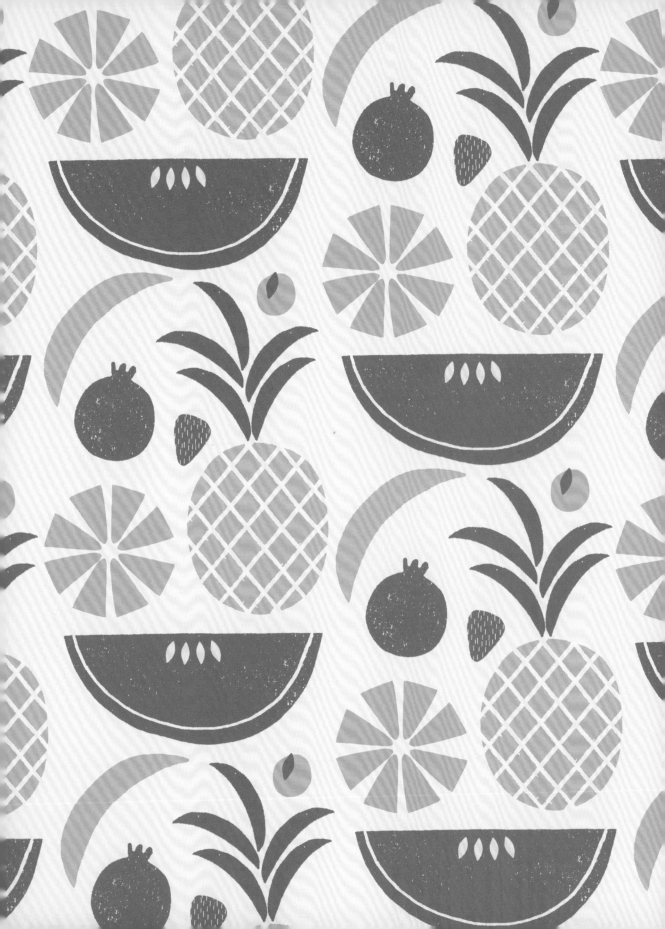

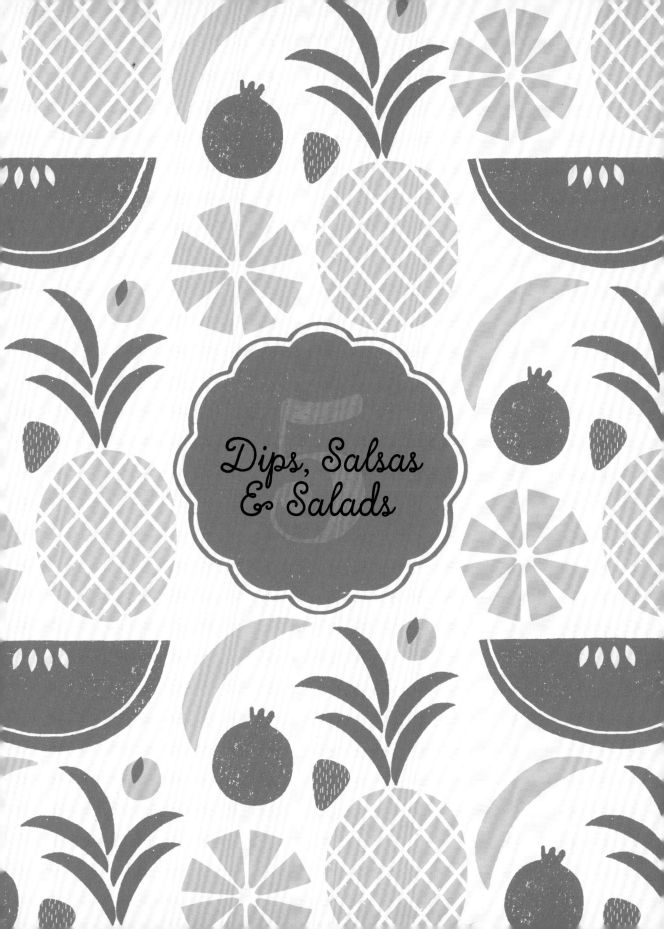

Dips, Salsas
& Salads

This selection of dips, salsas and salads can accompany main meals and they are also a great addition when entertaining or eating al fresco.

We enjoy eating together as a family and love having barbecues and picnics with friends in the summer. We wanted to put together some easy recipes that will help make these occasions worry-free from a food allergy perspective.

Sometimes the simplest meal can be turned into something really exciting with the addition of a dip or salsa. They are very quick to make and are good accompaniments to a grilled piece of meat or fish. Most of the salsa ingredients are things you would typically have in your fridge or salad bowl so it is always easy to rustle something up at the last minute.

The salads in this chapter are ones we make regularly for many different occasions. They make great lunchbox fillers for school or picnics and are great if you are entertaining family and friends at a barbecue. All the recipes can be increased to make larger quantities for entertaining and most of them can be prepared in advance, making life easier if you're cooking for a crowd.

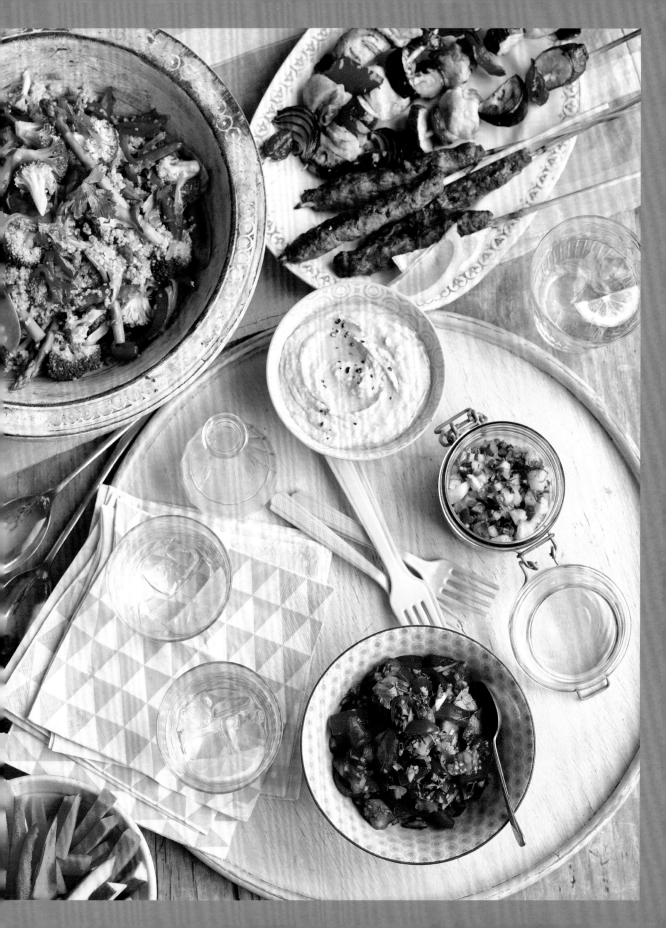

PREP: 10 MINUTES
COOK: NONE

This is a traditional Middle Eastern dip that is popular with kids and normally off-limits for those with sesame allergy. Our recipe has been adapted to taste just as good without the addition of tahini, a sesame paste, which is normally found in hummus. If you want to take this recipe a step further, you can add extra ingredients such as some ground coriander or roasted red peppers to give more variety of flavour.

HUMMUS

400g tin chickpeas,
    rinsed and drained
2 teaspoons ground
    cumin
1 garlic clove, peeled
Juice of 1 lemon
4 tablespoons olive oil
Freshly ground black
    pepper

1 Put all the ingredients in a blender and blitz to a smooth paste – you may need to add a little water to get the right consistency.

2 You can keep the hummus in a sealed plastic tub for an extra day in the fridge.

> *If you are not allergic*
>
> 2 tablespoons of tahini can be added to this recipe. Tahini is a great source of calcium.

A traditional Mexican dip, which is great served with any Mexican food such as Chilli Con Carne (see page 54), but is also tasty as a dip with crisps or, as Cammie likes it, to accompany some grilled chicken. It is not difficult to make and is much nicer than shop-bought guacamole, which often contains dairy products.

Rustic GUACAMOLE

2 ripe avocados
1 tablespoon very finely chopped red onion (adjust to taste)
Juice of 1 lime
1 small garlic clove, crushed
1 small tomato, chopped into small chunks
Pinch chilli powder (optional)
Freshly ground black pepper

1 Cut open the avocados, scoop out the flesh and pop it into a blender. Blitz until smooth. Add the onion, lime and garlic and quickly blitz again. Alternatively, if you prefer a chunkier texture, simply mash the avocados with a fork.

2 Stir in the tomato and season. Add a little chilli powder if you like some heat.

3 Place a sheet of clingfilm directly on the surface of the guacamole, covering it all, and then pop in the fridge until you are ready to serve. This will stop the surface going brown, like an apple can when it is left exposed to the air. This is best eaten the same day but will keep for 1 day in the fridge.

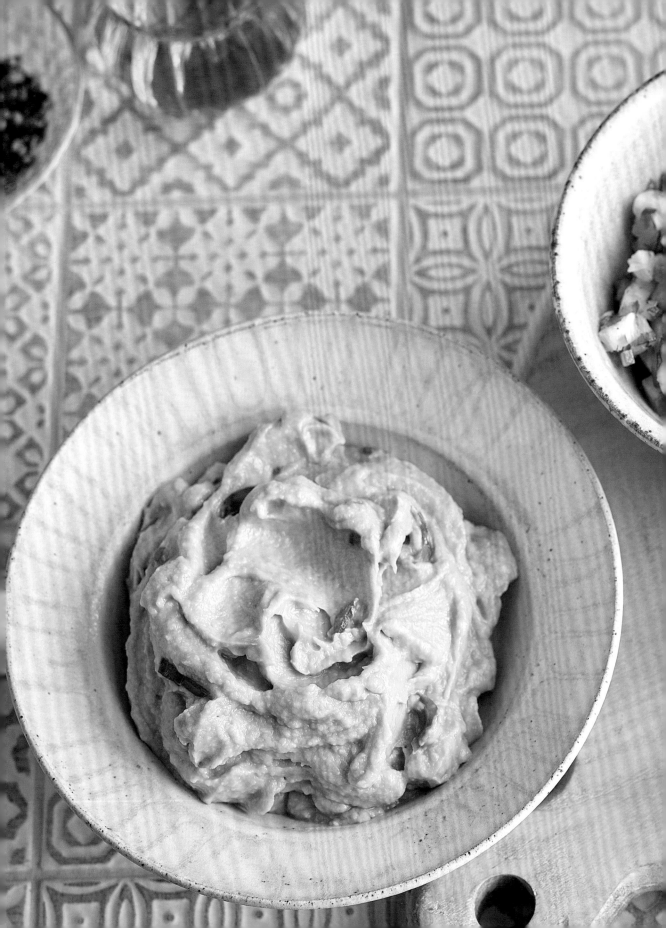

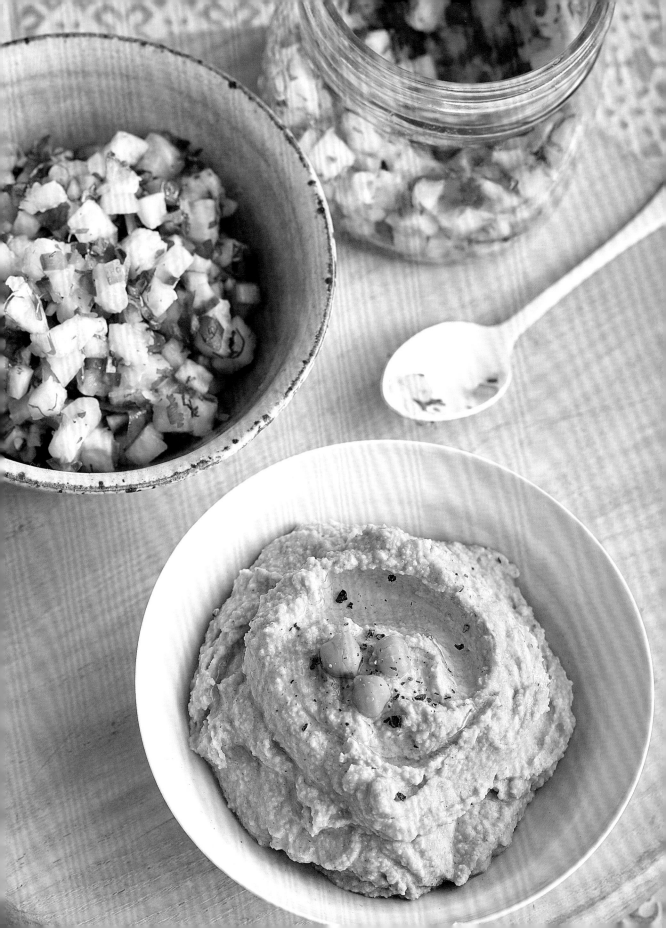

PREP: 10 MINUTES
COOK: NONE

Pineapple
SALSA

¼ red onion, finely
    chopped
½ fresh pineapple, peeled
    and finely diced
¼ cucumber, finely diced
¼ red pepper, deseeded
Handful fresh coriander,
    chopped
Handful fresh mint
    leaves, finely chopped
Juice of 1 lime
1 teaspoon olive oil

Fresh pineapple really is best for this but you can use tinned and it will still taste good. It is a colourful, fruity salsa that is great with grilled meat or oily fish. If you want a more grown-up flavour add a little fresh chopped chilli for a bit of heat. It is best eaten the same day as sometimes the colours can leach into each other if left for too long. A mandolin is great for creating small dice if you have one.

1 Put the onion in a sieve and pour over some boiling water – this will semi-cook the onion and take away the strong raw taste.

2 Combine the onion with all the remaining ingredients in a bowl and mix together.

....

Optional Extras
This also tastes great with the addition of diced mango.

SERVES A FAMILY OF 4

PREP: 10 MINUTES
COOK: NONE

Tomato SALSA

2 large tomatoes,
roughly diced
6 cherry tomatoes,
quartered
½ small red onion,
chopped
1 teaspoon finely chopped
fresh mint leaves
1 teaspoon chopped fresh
coriander leaves
Good squeeze of
lime juice

This salsa can be rustled up in moments and is great with so many dishes such as Homemade Beef Burgers (see page 116) or served with poppadoms and our Ever-so-Mild Chicken Korma (see page 110). You can make this a day in advance if needed, just cover and refrigerate.

1 Combine all the ingredients together in a bowl.

2 Store in an airtight container in the fridge for 1 day if not using straight away.

SERVES A FAMILY OF 4

PREP: 10 MINUTES
COOK: NONE

Cucumber SALSA

1 teaspoon finely
chopped shallot
½ cucumber, finely diced
(use a mandolin if you
have one)
2 teaspoons chopped
fresh coriander leaves
1 teaspoon chopped
fresh mint leaves
Juice of ½ small lemon
2 tablespoons olive oil

Cool and refreshing, Casper loves this salsa with Lamb Kebabs (see page 118). Make a few hours ahead and keep chilled in the fridge.

1 Put the shallot in a sieve and pour over some boiling water – this will semi-cook it and take away the strong raw taste.

2 Combine the shallot with all the other ingredients in a bowl and serve.

3 Store in an airtight container in the fridge for 1 day if not using straight away.

SERVES A FAMILY OF 4

PREP: 5 MINUTES
COOK: 1 HOUR

This is basically an aubergine purée that is eaten in many Mediterranean countries such as Greece, Turkey and Morocco. It's a lovely dip, perfect with crackers or as an accompaniment to meat or fish. It does take a little while to roast the aubergines but once that is done it is very quick to assemble.

AUBERGINE DIP

2 aubergines
2 garlic cloves, left
  whole with skin on
2 tablespoons olive oil
Squeeze of lemon juice
Sprinkle of chopped
  fresh parsley
Freshly ground black
  pepper

1 Preheat the oven to 200°C/190°C fan/400°F/Gas mark 6.

2 Place the whole aubergines on a baking tray and put them in the oven for about 1 hour – add the whole garlic cloves to the baking tray for the last 10 minutes of cooking. Remove from the oven when the aubergines are soft.

3 Scoop out the flesh from inside the aubergine and squeeze the pulp from the garlic, discarding the skin. Leave to cool.

4 Place the cooled aubergine flesh, garlic, oil and lemon juice in a blender and blitz to a paste.

5 Season with black pepper and garnish with parsley.

6 Store in an airtight container in the fridge for 1 day if not using straight away.

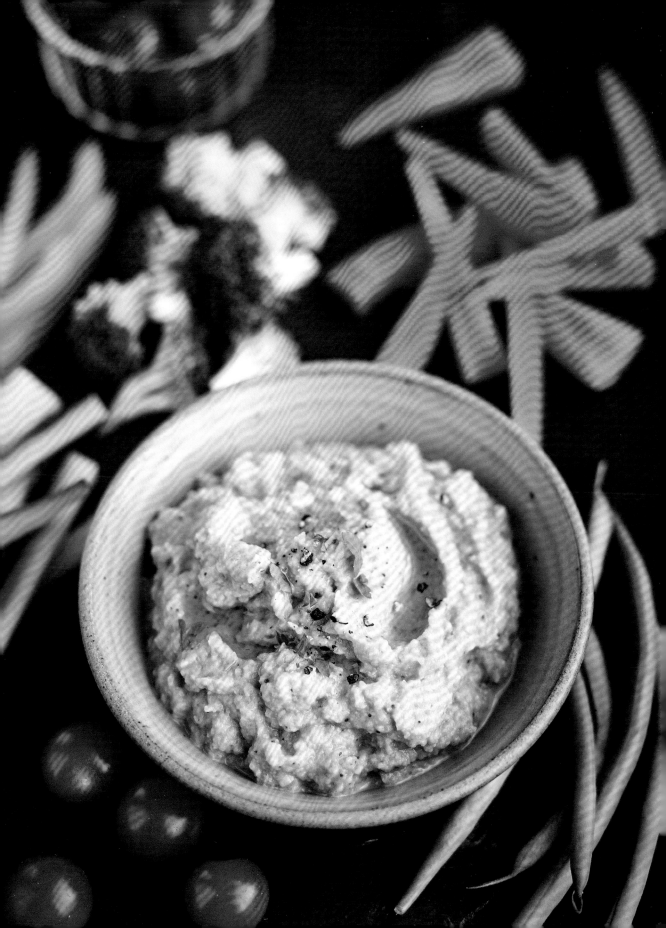

PREP: 10 MINUTES
COOK: NONE

CARROT
with Poppy Seeds

4 large carrots, peeled and coarsely grated
2 large tomatoes, cut into chunks
2 teaspoons poppy seeds
A handful watercress leaves (optional)

Dressing
2 tablespoons olive oil
1½ teaspoons cider vinegar

This is easy to rustle up in moments and makes a lovely side salad to go with a main meal or to serve at a barbecue.

1 Mix the carrots, tomatoes, poppy seeds and watercress, if using, in a bowl.

2 Mix the dressing ingredients together in a small bowl or jar and then pour over the salad before serving.

Optional Extras
Raisins can be added for a more fruity flavour.

PREP: 10 MINUTES
COOK: NONE

Tomato, Avocado and Basil SALAD

4 large tomatoes
2 avocados, cut in half, peeled and sliced
Good handful fresh basil leaves
Olive oil, for drizzling
Balsamic vinegar, for drizzling
Freshly ground black pepper

This is a really great combination that makes us think of summertime and is absolutely delicious especially when the tomatoes are lovely and ripe. This is very popular with all our children and goes well with any meat, and is, of course, very quick to prepare.

1 Slice the tomatoes and arrange on a plate, intermingled with slices of avocado.

2 Scatter basil leaves on top, season with black pepper and drizzle with oil and vinegar.

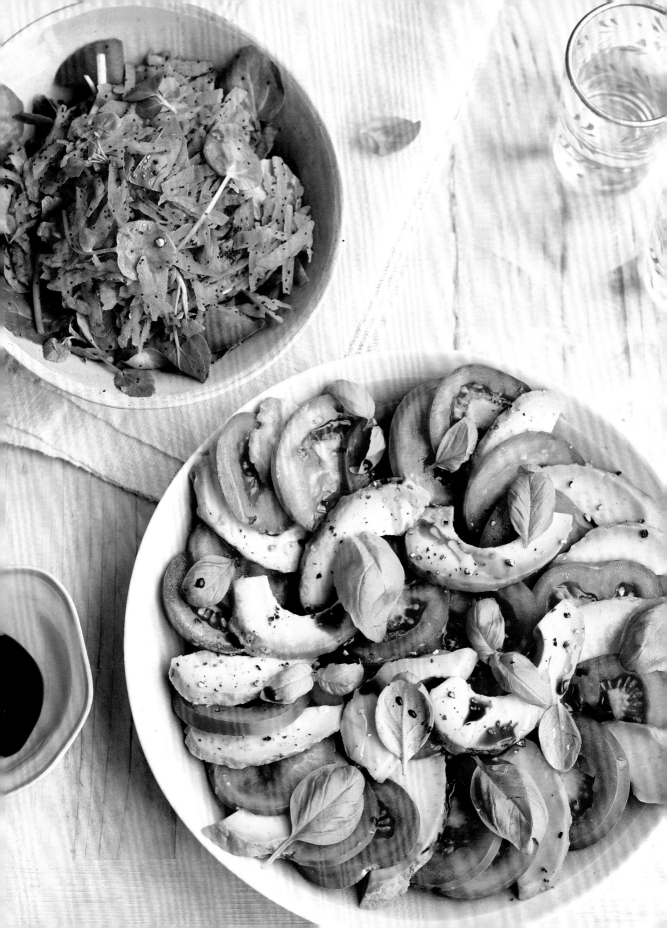

PREP: 10 MINUTES
COOK: NONE

The salad goes well with Jacket Potatoes (see page 192). You can use any variety of beans that you like – most supermarkets sell small tins of individual varieties of beans. You can also get tins of mixed beans for salads, which makes life easy. Make the salad a day ahead and keep chilled in the fridge.

Three Bean SALAD

200g tin cannellini
   beans, drained
   and rinsed
200g tin butter beans,
   drained and rinsed
Large handful fine
   green beans, cooked,
   chilled and chopped
Juice of 1 lemon
1 tablespoon chopped
   fresh parsley
1 garlic clove, crushed
1 tablespoon olive oil
Freshly ground black
   pepper

Combine all the ingredients in a bowl, season to taste and serve.

VARIATION
Add in a 125g tin of pilchards, sardines, tuna or mackerel.

SERVES
A FAMILY OF
4

PREP: 15 MINUTES
COOK: 25 MINUTES

A staple at barbecues, rice salad is always popular and particularly tasty if you try and keep an equal balance of rice to the other ingredients. If you want to make larger quantities just increase the main recipe and add the dressing as required. This is also a good, filling lunchbox option. Make a day ahead and keep chilled in the fridge.

RICE SALAD

160g long-grain rice
60g wild rice
Good handful frozen peas
1 red pepper, deseeded
  and diced
½ cucumber, chopped
  into small dice
5 sun-dried tomatoes,
  chopped
½ red onion, very
  finely chopped
Handful fresh parsley,
  finely chopped
Handful fresh basil
  leaves, finely chopped

Dressing
3 tablespoons olive oil
1 tablespoon white wine
  vinegar

1 Cook the rice as per the instructions on the packets, drain well and leave to cool.

2 Boil the peas, then drain and cool them in some cold water – this will keep them a lovely vibrant green colour. Drain once cold.

3 Put the rice, peas and the remaining ingredients together in a bowl. Mix the ingredients for the dressing together in a small bowl or jar.

4 Pour the dressing over the salad and serve immediately or chill in the fridge until needed (it will keep for 1 day in the fridge).

Optional Extras
This salad is a good base to add any other vegetables that you like – roasted vegetables are a good option. Also you can add cooked puy lentils or quinoa to make a more substantial salad.

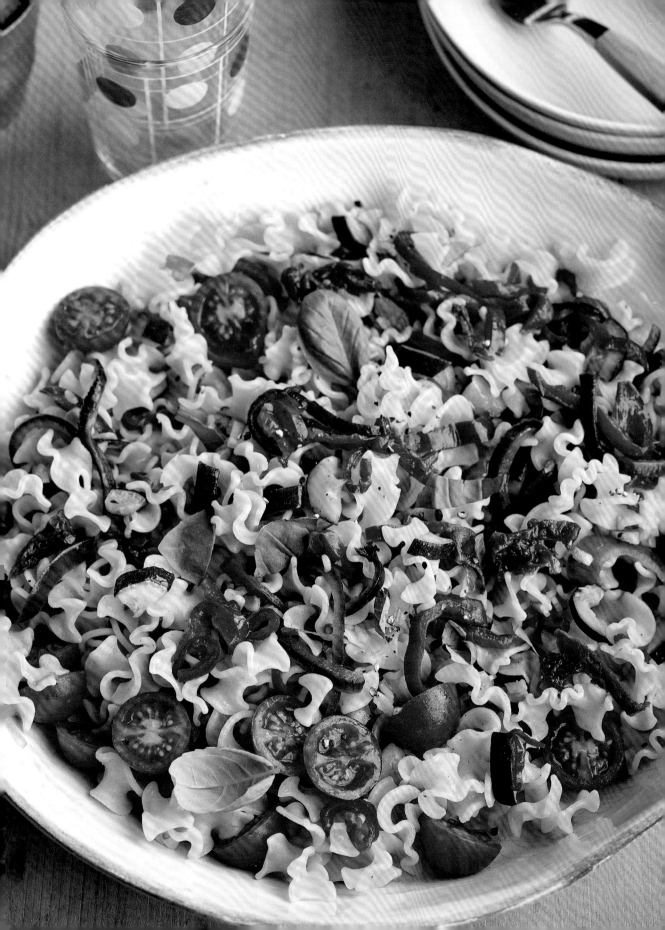

SERVES A FAMILY OF **4**

PREP: 10 MINUTES
COOK: 45 MINUTES

This is a pretty familiar salad that is often found in school lunchboxes or at summer parties. It is exceptionally easy to make and is a lovely filling salad on its own or as a side dish. It is also a great way to use up any leftover vegetables. When using gluten-free pasta, this salad is definitely best eaten the same day but it is possible to make a day ahead and then keep chilled in the fridge.

Colourful GLUTEN-FREE PASTA SALAD

1 courgette, quartered lengthways and sliced

½ red onion, sliced

1 red pepper, deseeded and finely sliced

Good drizzle of olive oil

225g dried gluten-free pasta (penne or spirals look nice)

6 sun-dried tomatoes, chopped

10 cherry tomatoes, cut in half

Handful fresh basil, roughly torn

Freshly ground black pepper

Dressing

1 tablespoon finely chopped shallots

3 tablespoons olive oil

1 tablespoon white wine vinegar

1 Preheat the oven to 220°C/200°C fan/425°F/Gas mark 7.

2 Drizzle the courgette, onion and pepper with a little oil in a roasting tin and toss well so they have an even coating. Roast in the oven for about 35–45 minutes until they start to take on a little colour.

3 Meanwhile, cook the pasta as per the instructions on the packet and drain well. Combine the dressing ingredients in a small bowl or jar.

4 Combine the roasted vegetables and sun-dried tomatoes with the pasta while still warm, then pour over the dressing, and mix really well. Leave to cool and then add the cherry tomatoes and basil.

Optional Extras
Like the Rice Salad (see page 143) this is delicious as it is but you can add any extra vegetables you have to hand such as aubergines, yellow peppers, and sweetcorn or herbs such as parsley and oregano.

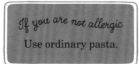

If you are not allergic
Use ordinary pasta.

PREP: 10 MINUTES
COOK: NONE

This is a fresh twist on traditional coleslaw as there is no mayonnaise. It is crunchy, fresh and delicious as a side dish to accompany a main meal. Make a day ahead and keep chilled in the fridge. Izzy and Casper both really like this.

Crunchy COLESLAW

¼ green cabbage, cut in half, hard core removed

¼ red cabbage, cut in half, hard core removed

1 large carrot, peeled and grated

4 radishes, very thinly sliced

Good handful fresh flat-leaf parsley, chopped

30g raisins

Freshly ground black pepper

Dressing
2 tablespoons olive oil
Juice of 1 lemon
1 teaspoon Dijon mustard (optional)

1 Shred the cabbage either by using a knife or a mandolin.

2 Combine all the ingredients in a bowl and mix well.

3 Mix the dressing in another bowl and add, combining all the ingredients together well.

> *If you are not allergic*
>
> Add in the optional mustard and mix in a little mayonnaise or salad cream on top of the dressing.

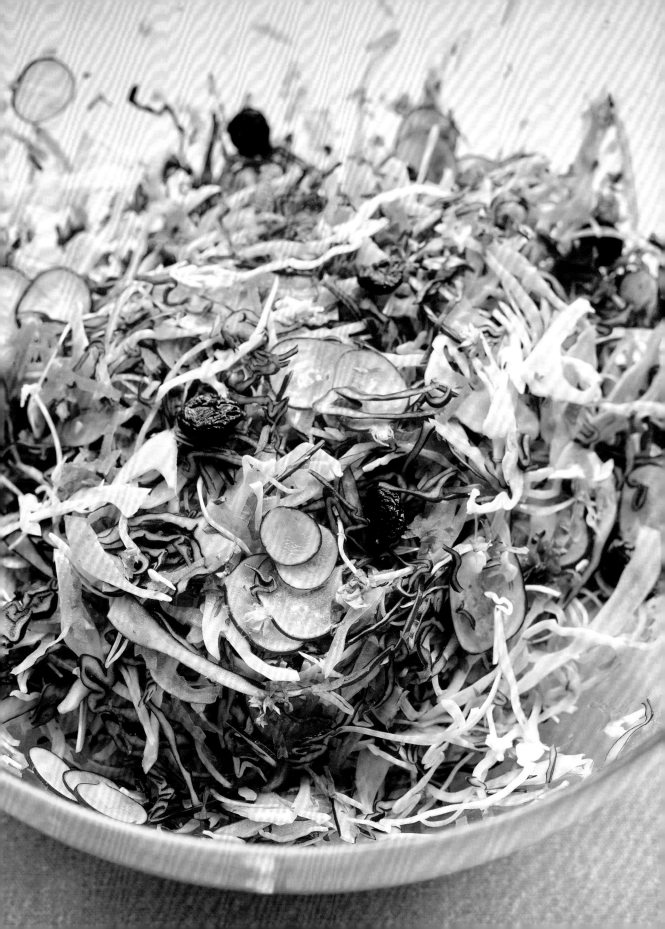

SERVES A FAMILY OF 4

PREP: 10 MINUTES
COOK: 30 MINUTES

This is a lovely cold salad dish but is also great served warm with a piece of grilled salmon or chicken. Make a day ahead and keep chilled in the fridge.

Puy LENTIL SALAD

100g Puy lentils
300ml water
1 teaspoon olive oil
1 small red pepper,
    deseeded and chopped
    into small pieces
2 celery sticks, chopped
    into small pieces
    (optional)
3 large garlic cloves,
    crushed
Handful frozen peas
Freshly ground black
    pepper

Dressing
3 tablespoons olive oil
1 tablespoon white
    wine vinegar
½ tablespoon lemon juice

1 Rinse the Puy lentils and cook according to the packet instructions.

2 Heat the olive oil in a small frying pan and gently cook the red pepper and celery, if using, for about 10 minutes, allowing them to soften.

3 Add the garlic and peas and cook for a further minute. Remove from the heat and set aside until the lentils are cooked.

4 Drain the lentils and add to the pan.

5 Combine the dressing ingredients in a small bowl. Pour over the salad, season to taste and mix well.

6 If serving hot, just heat a little more if needed. If serving as a salad, allow to cool and then serve.

VARIATION
If you would like to make the salad more substantial add 50g of cooked wild rice.

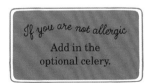
If you are not allergic
Add in the
optional celery.

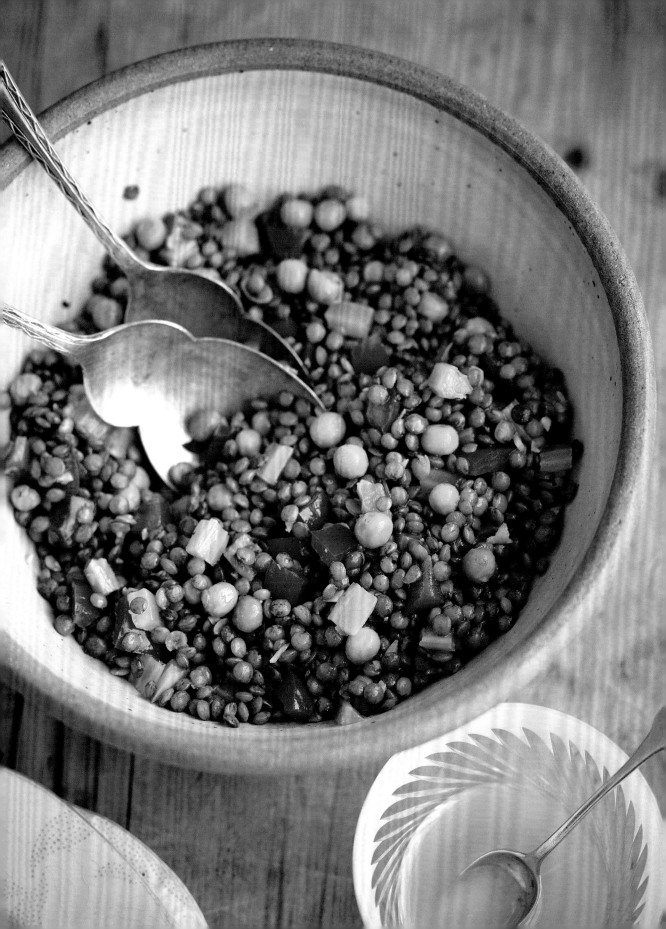

PREP: 10 MINUTES
COOK: 30 MINUTES

Some call quinoa (pronounced keen-wa) a superfood as it is a great source of protein and has lots of other nutrients. This is a vibrant and green salad and although there is plenty of quinoa it does not dominate the dish. By plunging the cooked vegetables into cold water you stop the cooking process immediately, keeping the vegetables a bright green colour and ensuring they won't go soggy.

Green Vegetable and QUINOA SALAD

45g quinoa
135ml cold water
1 teaspoon olive oil
1 red pepper, deseeded
  and cut into slices
1 shallot, sliced finely
100g mange tout
1 broccoli head, cut
  into bite-size florets
2 good handfuls
  frozen peas (petit
  pois are best)
125g fine asparagus
  spears
Handful fresh flat-leaf
  parsley, chopped
1 tablespoon chopped
  fresh chives

Dressing
Juice of 1 lemon
3 tablespoons olive oil
Freshly ground black
  pepper

1 Place the quinoa in a saucepan with the water and bring to the boil. Reduce the heat to a simmer and cook for 20 minutes until all the water has been absorbed.

2 Meanwhile, heat the olive oil in a pan over a medium to high heat and gently cook the red pepper, allowing it to soften and take on a little colour.

3 Add the shallot to the pan and cook for a minute or so, just until the shallot has softened, and then set aside.

4 Bring a large pan of water to the boil and then add all the green vegetables. Allow the water to come back to the boil and cook the vegetables for about 30 seconds. It may be easier to cook the vegetables in batches depending on the size of your pan.

5 Drain the vegetables and plunge them immediately into cold water – you may need to change the water a few times to keep it cold.

6 When the vegetables are cold, drain and set aside.

7 To assemble the salad, toss the vegetables, quinoa, parsley, chives and dressing ingredients together in a bowl and chill in the fridge before serving.

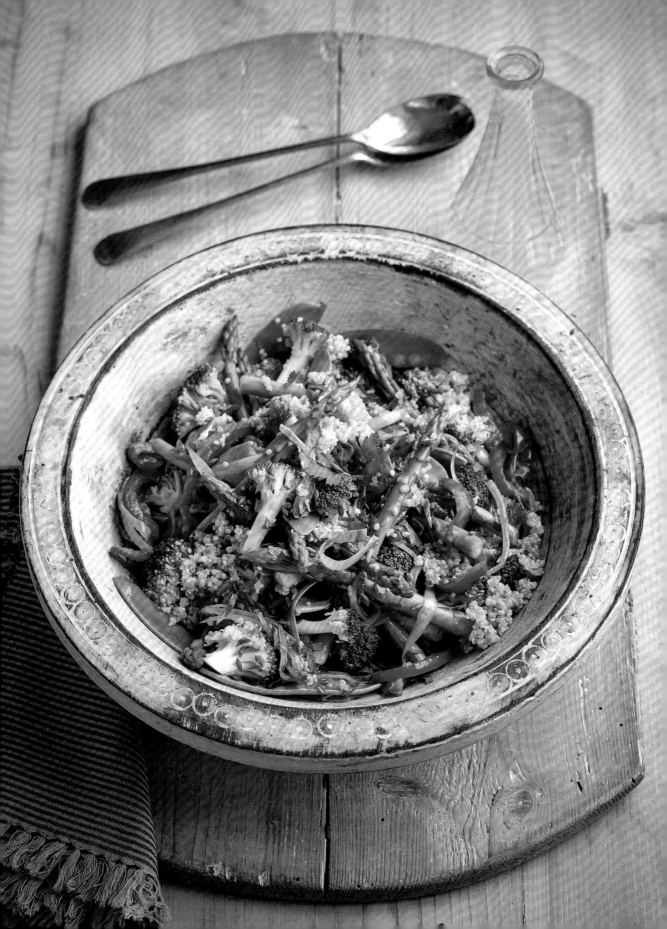

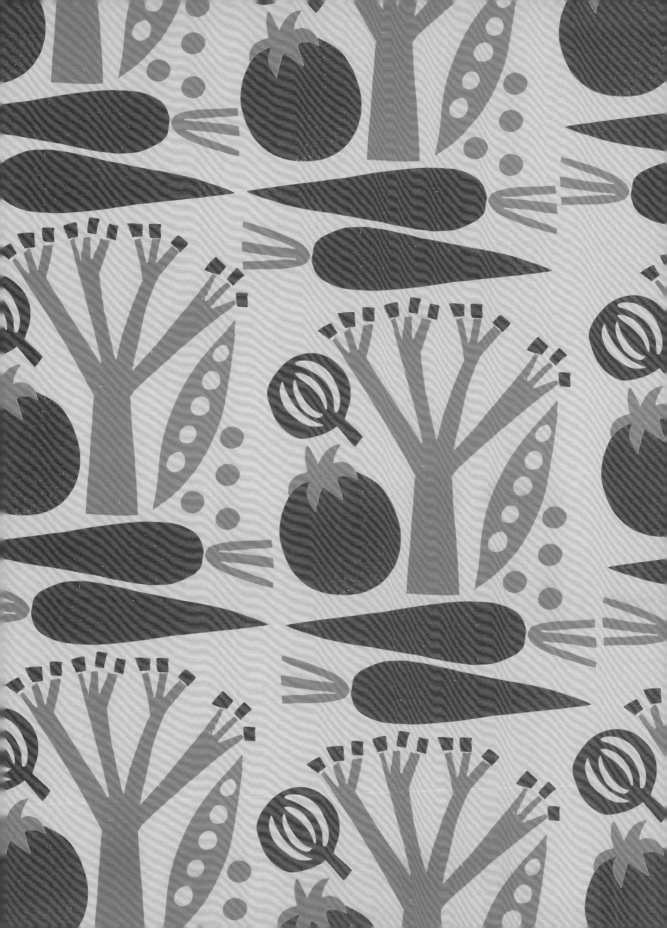

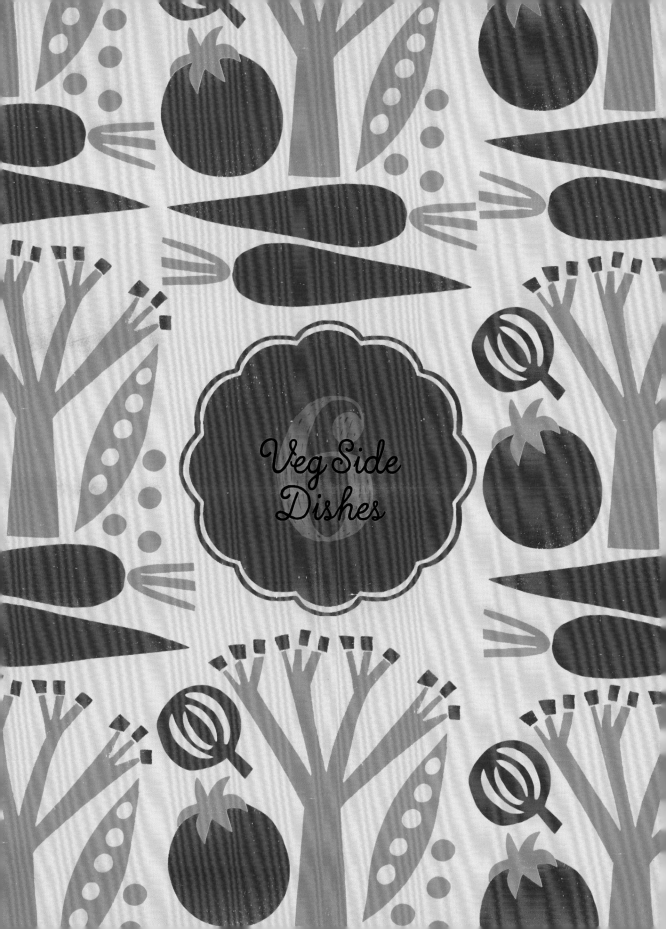

6

Veg Side
Dishes

There are so many varieties of vegetables available in shops these days, and they can all be prepared in many different ways, ensuring there is always something you can give even the fussiest of eaters. If you have a child who is not keen on their vegetables try our Five-a-Day Pasta Sauce (see page 42), which has lots of vegetables blended through it but has a nice sweet taste. You can also disguise vegetables in casseroles and other one-pot dishes. Do also try our Peas with Bacon (see page 158) and Sweet Roasted Carrots with Garlic and Coriander (see page 167) as they tend to be popular too.

It's a good idea to provide lots of variety and serve a broad range of vegetables to get different vitamins and nutrients. Depending on the allergy, your child's dietitian can help you identify those vitamins your child may need. In many countries across the world it is recommended that adults and children should eat at least five portions of fruit and vegetables every day. The benefits of eating them daily are well documented and if your child can eat at least five portions each day this will help maintain a balanced diet.

You can steam, boil, microwave and roast most vegetables very successfully. Steaming is a good option as it tends to preserve more nutrients than other cooking methods. However if you have a bit more time and want to make the vegetables more interesting, this chapter offers a selection of tasty and somewhat more adventurous vegetable side dishes.

All our vegetable side dishes are designed to serve a family of four as an accompaniment to a main meal but you can adjust quantities to suit your family.

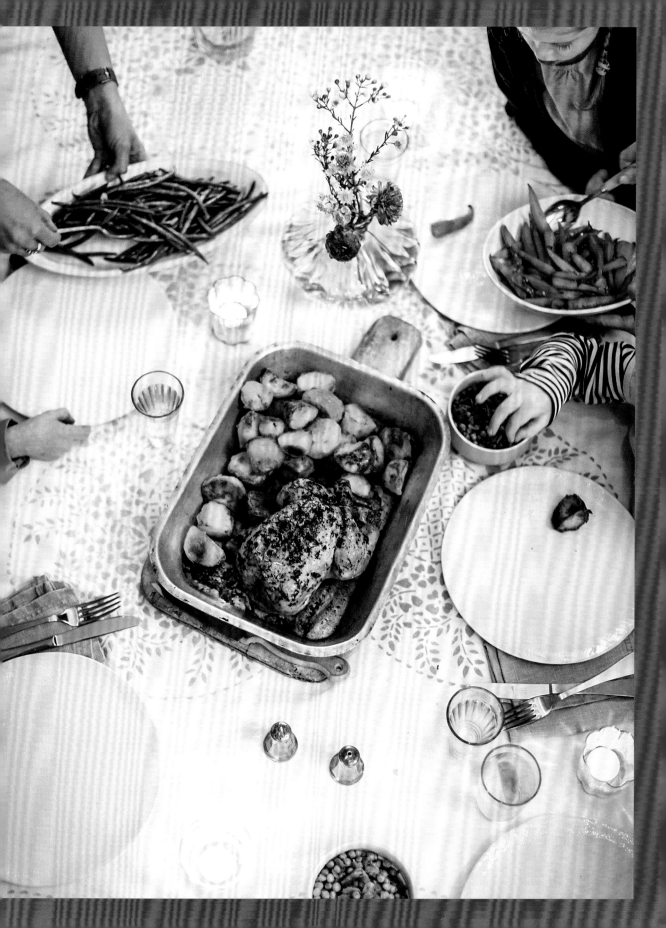

SERVES A FAMILY OF 4

PREP: 5 MINUTES
COOK: 15 MINUTES

We eat this a lot for breakfast, but with a little less garlic. It is a lovely side or simple supper dish on its own with crackers or a hunk of your favourite free-from bread.

GARLIC MUSHROOMS
with Lemon and Parsley

1 tablespoon olive oil
3 garlic cloves, crushed
675g mushrooms, chopped (chestnut, button, Portobello are all suitable)
Juice of ½ lemon
50ml fresh Vegetable Stock (see page 248) or just use boiling water
Handful fresh parsley, chopped

1 Heat the oil in a large frying pan and add the garlic and the mushrooms (don't worry if it looks a lot as they reduce down quickly). Cook for about 10 minutes over a medium to high heat, stirring occasionally.

2 Pour over the lemon juice, stock or water, stir well and cook for about 5 minutes or until the mushrooms are tender and the liquid has reduced. If the mushrooms are cooked before the liquid has reduced, remove the mushrooms, rapidly boil the liquid and then pour back over the mushrooms.

3 Sprinkle with parsley and serve.

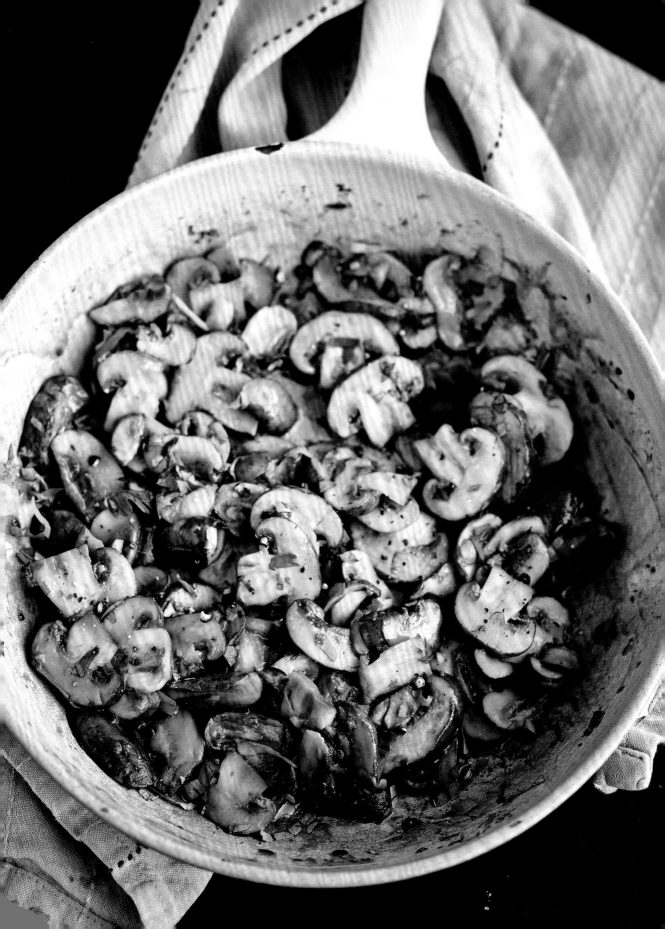

FINE GREEN BEANS
with Olive Oil and Garlic

SERVES A FAMILY OF 4

PREP: 5 MINUTES
COOK: 5 MINUTES

200g fine green beans
Olive oil, for drizzling
1 large garlic clove,
    crushed
Freshly ground black
    pepper

If you are not allergic

Add a small handful of
sliced almonds during
the last stage.

By just adding a little bit of garlic and oil to the green beans they look lovely and glossy and taste delicious. Izzy isn't very fond of green beans generally but she does like them cooked like this.

1 Bring a saucepan of water to the boil. Add the green beans, cook until tender, drain, and return to the pan.

2 Toss in a little olive oil, stir in the garlic and cook over a low heat for a further minute or two.

SERVES A FAMILY OF 4

PREP: 5 MINUTES
COOK: 10 MINUTES

PEAS
with Bacon

4 streaky bacon rashers,
    finely chopped
2 teaspoons very finely
    chopped shallots
    or onions
350g frozen peas

This is a really tasty combination of ingredients that most children seem to like. Peas tend to be popular on their own but with the addition of bacon they are even better. This is one of Casper's favourites.

1 Fry the bacon in a frying pan over a medium heat in its own fat until lovely and crispy.

2 Add the shallots and peas and cook for 5 more minutes.

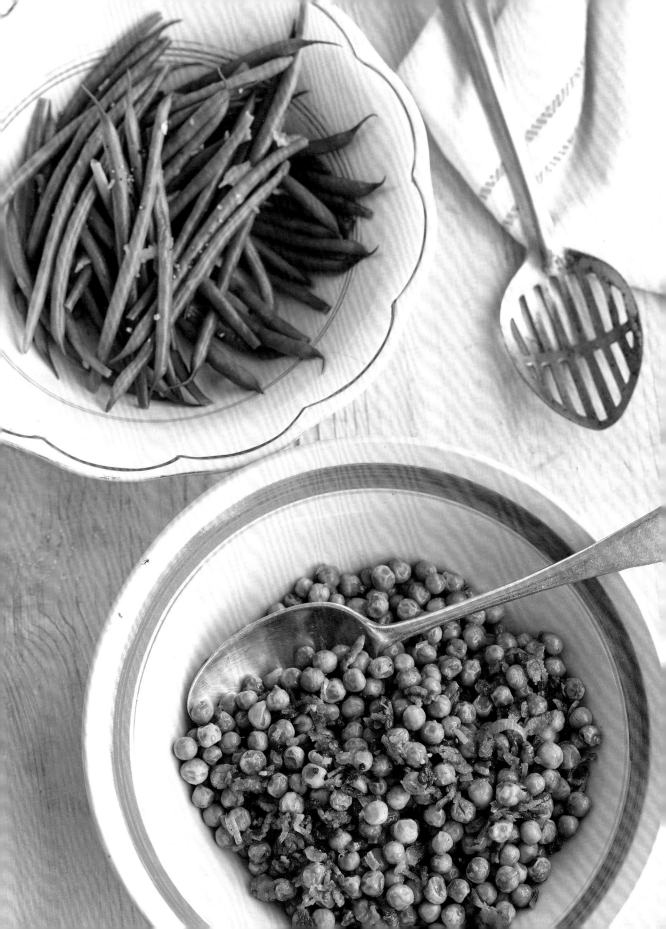

SERVES
A FAMILY OF
4

PREP: 5 MINUTES
COOK: 10 MINUTES

Our kids love spinach on its own, just simply wilted in the pan. But sometimes it is nice to make it more interesting with some lovely aromatic spices. It only takes a few moments longer to make but is definitely worth it.

aromatic SPINACH

1 teaspoon olive oil
1 small shallot,
   finely chopped
1 garlic clove, crushed
1 teaspoon ground
   coriander
2 teaspoons whole
   cumin seeds
300g spinach, washed

1 Heat the oil in a large frying pan over a low heat and gently fry the shallot for about 3 minutes until softened.

2 Add the garlic, coriander and cumin and stir well.

3 Add the spinach, stir and allow to wilt in the pan.

SERVES A FAMILY OF 4

PREP: 5 MINUTES
COOK: 10 MINUTES

This is a recipe that is traditionally made after a Christmas dinner to use up leftover Brussels sprouts and roast potatoes. However, it is great with any cooked potatoes and at any time of the year. Any leftover vegetables can be added if your kids are not keen on sprouts – just use roughly equal quantities of potato and vegetables. Casper will sometimes request this for breakfast.

BUBBLE AND SQUEAK

1 tablespoon olive oil
350g Roast Potatoes
   (see page 178),
   cooked, cooled and
   roughly chopped
350g Brussels sprouts,
   cooked, cooled and
   roughly chopped
Freshly ground black
   pepper

1 Heat the oil in a large frying pan and fry the potatoes and Brussels Sprouts until they are golden brown. Add a little extra oil if needed.

2 Season with black pepper and serve.

SERVES A FAMILY OF 4

PREP: 10 MINUTES
COOK: 1 HOUR

This is so easy and great with grilled or barbecued meat and fish, or even with a Sunday roast. You can use any combination of vegetables that you like but it is nice to have a variety of colour. This side dish is good to make if you are having people over or are busy. It can be prepared in advance and is then very happy in the oven with little attention.

Mediterranean ROASTED VEGETABLES

½ red pepper, deseeded and chopped
½ yellow pepper, deseeded and chopped
½ red onion, chopped
½ butternut squash, peeled and chopped
2 carrots, peeled and chopped
1 large courgette, chopped
1 aubergine, chopped
3 garlic cloves, left whole and unpeeled
2 tablespoons olive oil
2 fresh rosemary sprigs
Freshly ground black pepper

1 Preheat the oven to 220°C/200°C fan/425°F/Gas mark 7.

2 Pop all the vegetables into a large baking tray, drizzle with the olive oil and scatter over the rosemary.

3 Roast for about 1 hour until the vegetables are cooked and lightly browned at the edges.

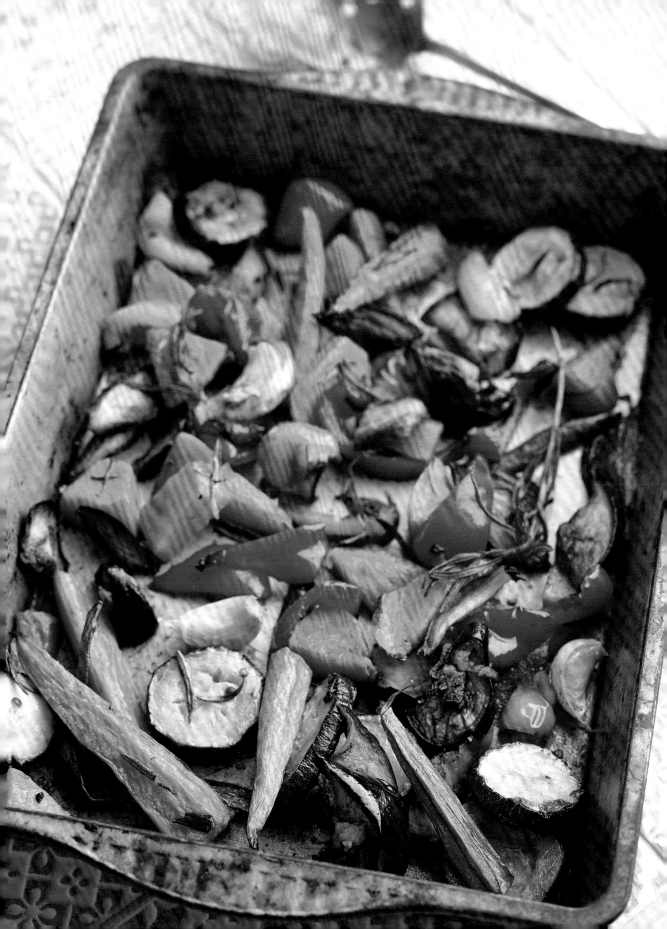

PREP: 10 MINUTES
COOK: 2 HOURS

This is a lovely winter dish and so good with roast pork and mashed potato. This recipe is made using a third of an average red cabbage but if you have a large casserole dish increase the quantities to cook the entire cabbage and freeze in batches. This can also be made the day before and then reheated.

RED CABBAGE

300g red cabbage, stalk
    removed and shredded
120g cooking apple,
    core removed, peeled
    and chopped
100g onion, finely
    chopped
½ garlic clove, crushed
1 tablespoon redcurrant
    jelly, from a jar
1 tablespoon brown sugar
1 tablespoon white
    wine vinegar
Freshly ground black
    pepper

1 Preheat the oven to 160°C/140°C fan/325°F/Gas mark 3.

2 Add all the ingredients to a large ovenproof pan or casserole and place a lid on top.

3 Cook in the oven for about 2 hours, stirring occasionally. If at any time you feel it is starting to look dry, add a little water to the pan.

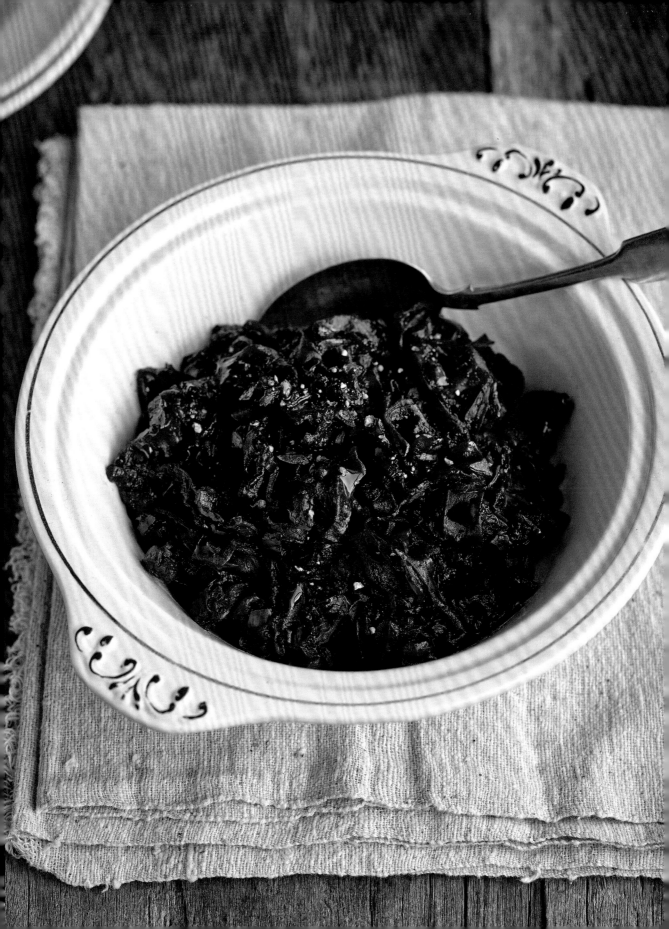

PREP: 10 MINUTES
COOK: 1 HOUR

A traditional Southern French vegetable stew, this is great as a topping for our Jacket Potatoes (see page 192) or as a side with a piece of grilled chicken. This is easy to make a day in advance; just cook, leave to cool, cover, chill and reheat fully when needed. It will also freeze well, although be aware that when defrosted and reheated it can be a little softer than before.

RATATOUILLE

1 tablespoon olive oil
1 red pepper, chopped
    into chunks
1 large red onion,
    roughly chopped
1 aubergine, chopped
    into chunks
2 large courgettes,
    chopped into chunks
1 beef or very large
    tomato, chopped
    into chunks
200ml tomato passata
Freshly ground black
    pepper

1 Preheat the oven to 220°C/200°C fan/425°F/Gas mark 7.

2 Put the oil, red pepper, onion, aubergine and courgettes in a large roasting tin, moving the vegetables around so they're coated in the oil.

3 Roast for about 50 minutes in the oven until the vegetables start to take on a little colour at the edges.

4 Add the tomato, passata and some black pepper and return to the oven for a further 10 minutes.

5 Give everything a good stir before serving.

PREP: 5 MINUTES
COOK: 30 MINUTES

Carrot and coriander is a classic combination of flavours. This recipe is great with small, sweet Chantenay carrots but it is very nice with ordinary carrots too – just peel and chop them into sticks. The roasted carrots are sweet and sticky with an intense flavour and kids always seem to want second helpings. Zara is a big fan of these.

SWEET ROASTED CARROTS
with Garlic and Coriander

500g small Chantenay carrots or ordinary carrots chopped into sticks

1 tablespoon olive oil

1 large garlic clove, crushed

1 teaspoon coriander seeds

1 tablespoon runny honey (or maple syrup if you prefer)

1 Preheat the oven to 220°C/200°C fan/425°F/Gas mark 7.

2 Drizzle the carrots with the oil in a roasting tin and place in the oven for 10 minutes.

3 Combine the remaining ingredients in a bowl and then add them to the roasting tin with the carrots. Return to the oven for a further 30 minutes until the carrots are tender and have a lovely golden colour and glaze.

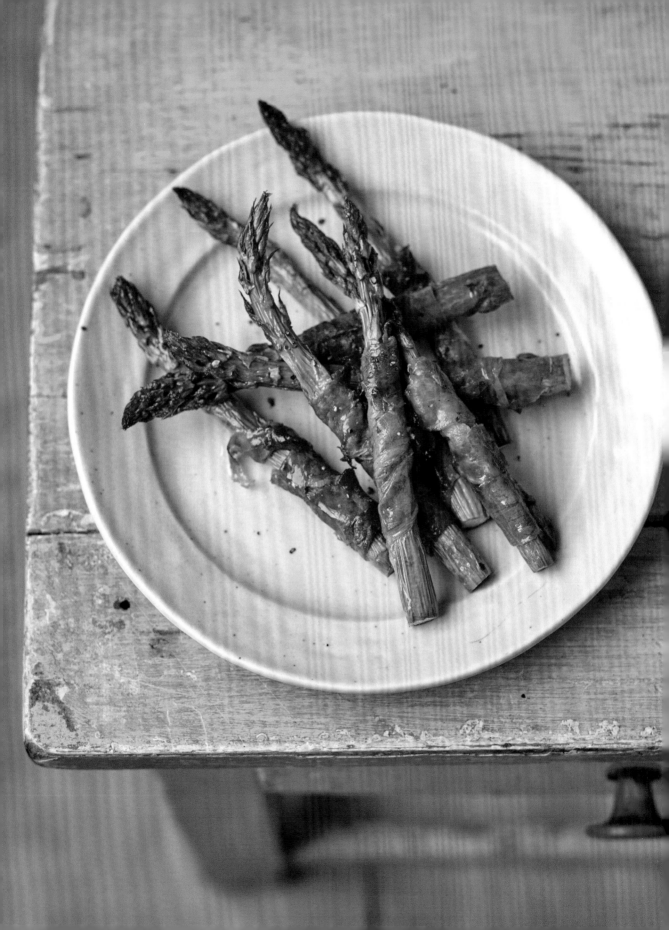

PREP: 5 MINUTES
COOK: 15 MINUTES

This has to be one of the simplest combinations and it is great as a side dish or as an easy starter at parties. The asparagus can also be cooked on the barbecue.

ASPARAGUS
with Prosciutto Ham

16 asparagus spears
8 prosciutto ham slices
Olive oil, for drizzling

1 Preheat the oven to 220°C/200°C fan/425°F/Gas mark 7.

2 Snap off the woody ends of the asparagus. Wrap a piece of ham around the middle of each asparagus. If your asparagus is very thin you may wish to bundle more spears together.

3 Place the asparagus on a baking tray and just drizzle the tips with a little olive oil. You don't need to put any oil on the ham.

4 Roast in the oven for about 10–15 minutes until the asparagus is tender and the prosciutto ham lovely and crispy.

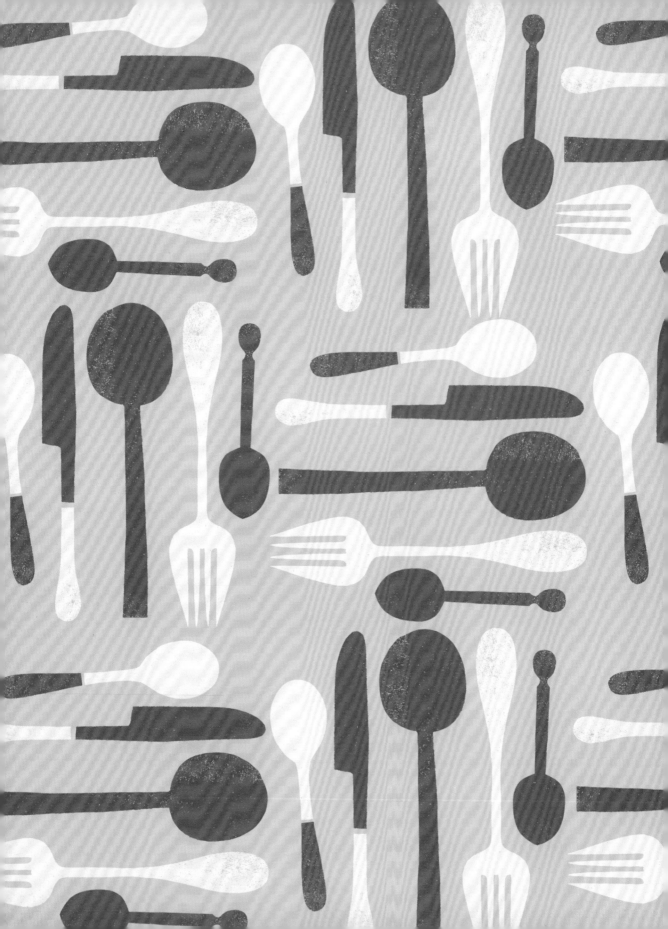

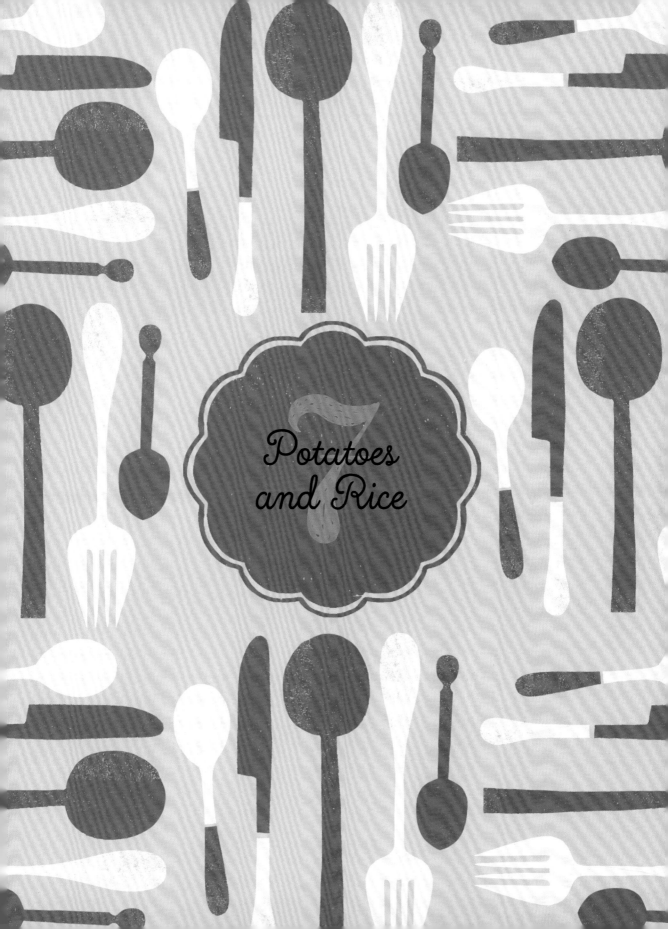

7

Potatoes and Rice

If your child is on a gluten-free diet they will need to get carbohydrates into their diet by eating more rice and potatoes, so it is essential to keep them interesting and enticing. Carbohydrates are important for providing energy and should form part of every meal alongside a source of protein such as meat or fish, plus vegetables or fruit.

Of course, there are lots of easy wins when it comes to potatoes that kids always love, such as oven chips and jacket potatoes, but it is nice to have more variety, especially if you are eating together as a family. Here, we have given you easy recipes to turn the humble potato into something delicious and different every night of the week.

Rice is also very easy to cook with many different varieties available to buy: long-grain, basmati, Thai jasmine, camargue red rice and wild rice. The easiest way to cook rice is by boiling it in a saucepan with plenty of water – always check the instructions on the packet for cooking times.

As with other grains it is possible to buy both white and whole grain brown rice. Brown rice is considered to be a healthier choice as it has more nutrients and fibre than refined white rice. Just remember to check the cooking times on the packet as it can take longer to cook.

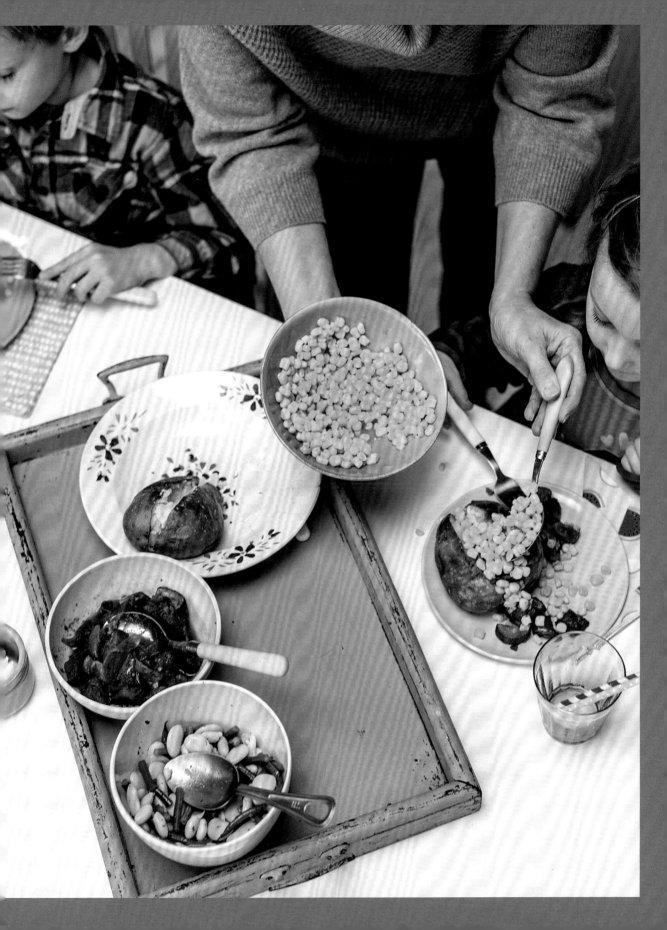

These are oven baked, sliced potatoes that are cooked in stock and flavoured with rosemary. Once you have sliced and layered up the potatoes, it is so easy to pop them in the oven and let them cook on their own while you get on with other things. We often serve these potatoes when we have friends over for lunch and if you're making large quantities, it speeds things up to use a mandolin as well to achieve consistently thin slices. If you want to get ahead, simply assemble the entire dish and chill so you can cook it when you are ready – just increase the cooking time a little if cooking straight from the fridge.

SERVES A FAMILY OF 4

PREP: 15 MINUTES
COOK: 50 MINUTES

Boulangère POTATOES

750g floury potatoes, such as Desiree, peeled and finely sliced
1 small onion, sliced as finely as you can
2 fresh rosemary sprigs, leaves chopped
750ml fresh Vegetable Stock (see page 248) or ½ vegetable stock from cube (!) dissolved in 750ml boiling water
Olive oil, for drizzling
Freshly ground black pepper

1 Preheat the oven to 220°C/200°C fan/425°F/Gas mark 7.

2 Place a layer of potatoes across the base of an ovenproof dish, then add a sprinkle of sliced onion, a grind of black pepper and then a sprinkle of rosemary.

3 Keep layering up the dish with potatoes, onions and seasoning and make the last layer just potato.

4 Pour the stock over everything until it comes to just under the top layer of potatoes (the amount needed will depend on the size of your dish). Top up with water if necessary.

5 Drizzle a little oil on top and bake in the oven for 50–60 minutes until the top layer of potatoes is golden brown and all the potatoes are cooked through.

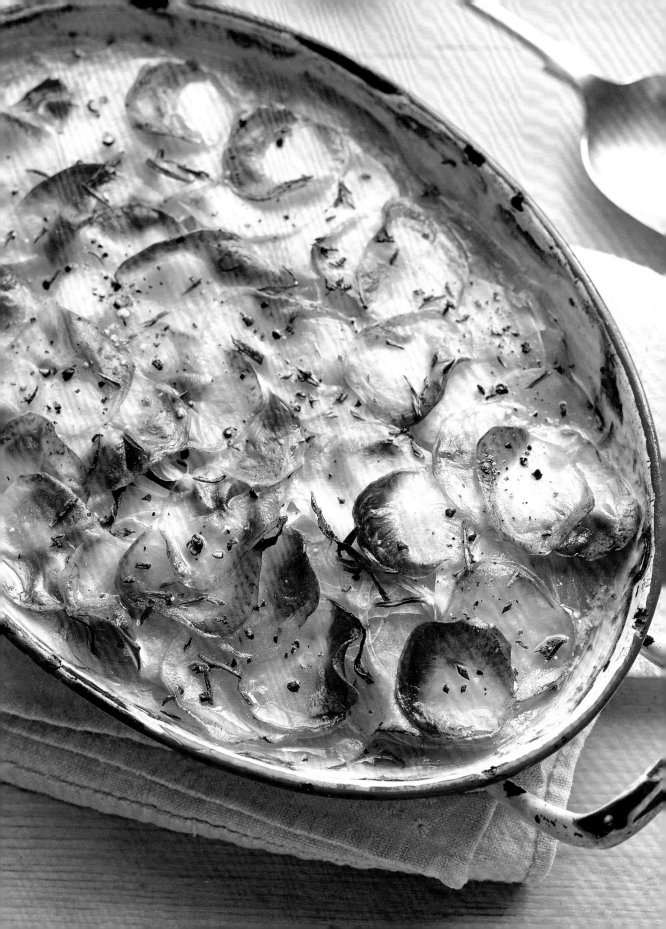

SERVES
A FAMILY OF
4

PREP: 10 MINUTES
COOK: 25 MINUTES

These are pan-fried discs of potato cooked with slices of onion. As they cook the potatoes become lovely and crispy around the edges and the onions become slightly sweet and caramelised.

Lyonnaise POTATOES

500g floury potatoes,
   such as Maris Piper,
   peeled and sliced into
   discs about ½ cm thick
Good splash sunflower oil
1½ onions, sliced
2 tablespoons chopped
   fresh parsley
Freshly ground black
   pepper

1 Boil the potatoes in a saucepan of water for a few minutes so they are just tender and then drain. Leave to cool slightly while you cook the onions.

2 Heat a little of the oil in a large frying pan over a medium heat and slowly cook the onions for about 10 minutes so they brown nicely but don't burn them. Remove the onions from the pan and set aside.

3 Add a little more oil to the pan and fry the par-boiled potatoes. Don't overload the pan or they won't brown – you may need to do this in batches.

4 Put all the potatoes and onions back into the pan for a further minute, sprinkle with the parsley and season with black pepper.

MAKES

8

PREP: 45 MINUTES
COOK: 25 MINUTES

These are little rounds of grated potato that are formed into patties and pan fried. They take a bit of time as you need to wait for some of the moisture to come out of the potato but as they freeze so well it is worth making extra. Simply freeze the cooked and cooled rosti and then reheat from frozen in the oven when needed.

POTATO ROSTI

675g floury potatoes,
   such as Maris Piper,
   peeled and grated
Sunflower oil, for frying
1 onion, very finely sliced
Salt and freshly ground
   black pepper

1 Preheat the oven to 220°C/200°C fan/425°F/Gas mark 7.

2 Put the grated potatoes and a sprinkle of salt in a colander or sieve and leave it to sit over a bowl for 30 minutes – this will allow moisture to come out of the potatoes.

3 Heat a little oil in a frying pan over a medium to high heat, gently cook the onion for about 5 minutes until it is soft and set aside.

4 Squeeze the potato really well to remove any more excess moisture and then mix with the onion and season with pepper. Form the mixture into little pancake shapes or make one large rosti the size of your frying pan.

5 Heat a little oil in your largest ovenproof frying pan and add the little rostis or, if making a large one, pat down well to help it form a neat shape. You may need to fry these in batches if your pan is not big enough.

6 Fry for a couple of minutes over a medium heat, until the rosti have some nice colour and crispiness, then pop the pan in the oven for about 20 minutes or until they are golden brown all over.

7 Turn the rostis once during cooking, taking care that they keep their shape. Use a slice to help you. You can add a little more oil if you need it at this stage.

....

Optional extras
You can add one rasher of uncooked chopped bacon or other grated vegetables such as half a medium carrot or parsnip to the mixture before frying.

PREP: 5 MINUTES
COOK: 1¼ HOURS

Everyone loves roast potatoes, especially with a roast dinner, but they must be lovely and crispy on the outside and beautifully fluffy on the inside. We think this recipe makes the most perfect roast potatoes. We often make extra as they are great heated up the next day for Bubble and Squeak (see page 161).

Perfect ROAST POTATOES

750g floury potatoes,
   (Maris Piper are great),
   peeled and cut into
   large chunks
3 tablespoons
   sunflower oil

1 Preheat the oven to 220°C/200°C fan/425°F/Gas mark 7.

2 Boil the potatoes in a large saucepan of water until they are only just tender. Drain and shake the potatoes a little in the colander to bash the edges slightly as this will help them go lovely and crispy.

3 Leave the potatoes to cool a little. If they go straight into the oven still steaming this can prevent them from going crispy.

4 Pour the oil into a large roasting tin and put this in the oven to warm up.

5 Add the potatoes to the preheated roasting tin and cook for about 45–60 minutes, turning once or twice during cooking.

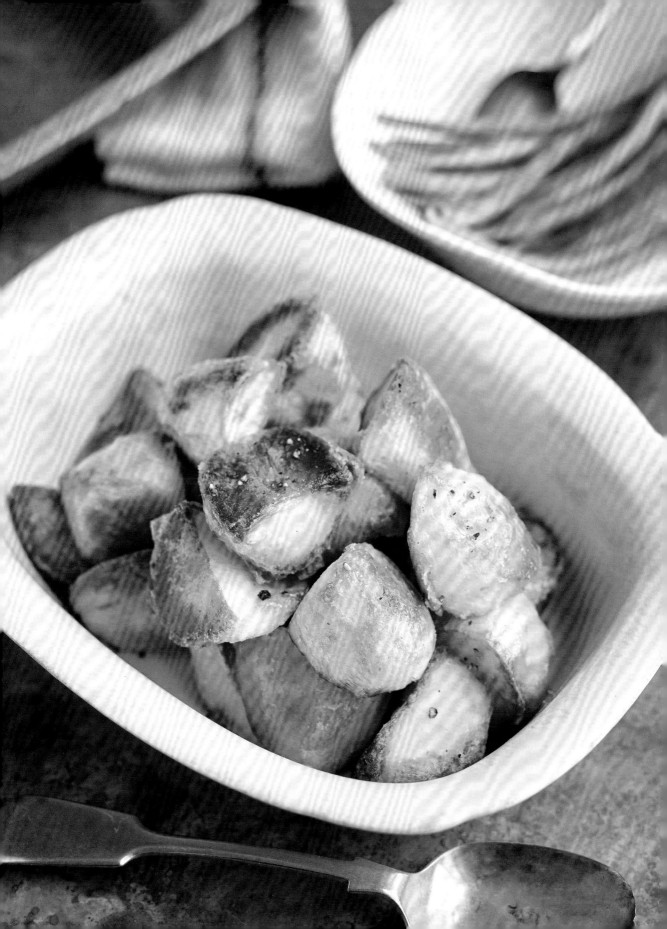

This is a great base recipe and the types of herbs and quantities can be adjusted to suit your personal taste. This potato salad is tasty and substantial in a lunchbox with a piece of cold meat or fish. It is a staple for us at family barbecues and can easily be made in advance.

Baby New POTATO SALAD

675g baby new potatoes, cut in half if they are large
2 tablespoons finely chopped fresh chives
1 tablespoon chopped fresh mint

Dressing
3 tablespoons olive oil
½ tablespoon white wine vinegar
½ tablespoon lemon juice
2 tablespoons finely chopped shallots
1 teaspoon grainy mustard (optional)

1 Boil the potatoes in a saucepan of water until just tender and then drain. This will take about 10 minutes depending on their size, but prod every so often with a fork to test.

2 Make the dressing by combining all the ingredients in a bowl and mixing well.

3 Pour the dressing over the potatoes while they are still warm and then leave to cool.

4 Add the herbs, toss well and serve.

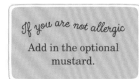

If you are not allergic
Add in the optional mustard.

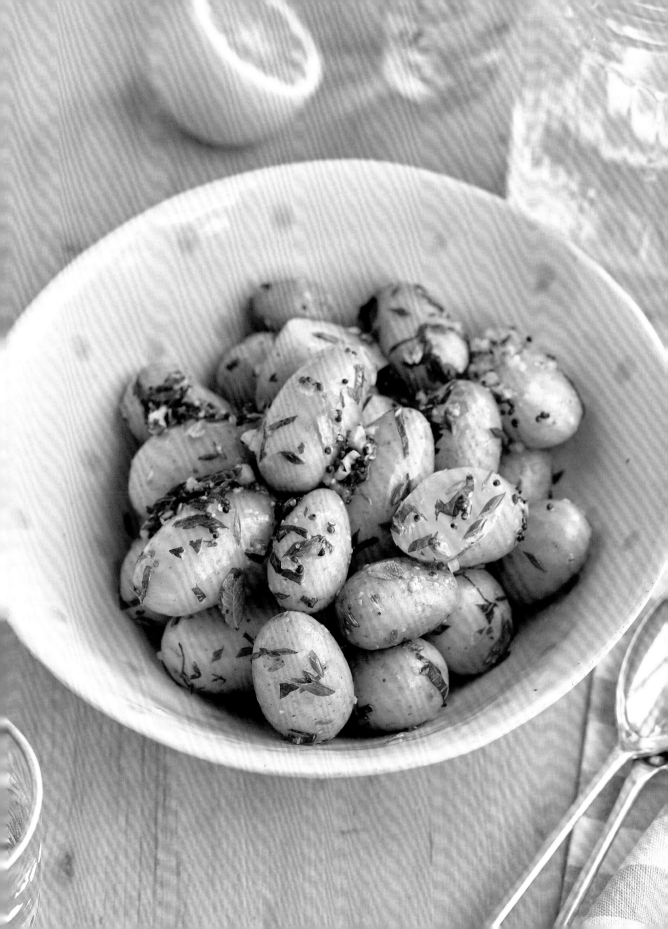

SERVES A FAMILY OF 4

PREP: 5 MINUTES
COOK: 20 MINUTES

Normally mash is off the menu for people with dairy allergy but adding a courgette to the mashed potato makes up for the lack of milk and butter. This recipe is also used to top our Shepherd's Pie (see page 115).

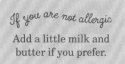

Mashed POTATO

1 tablespoon olive oil, plus extra to finish
1 shallot, finely chopped
900g floury potatoes, such as Maris Piper, peeled and chopped
1 courgette, sliced

If you are not allergic
Add a little milk and butter if you prefer.

1 Heat the oil in a saucepan over medium to high heat and fry the shallot for a couple of minutes until it has softened.

2 Add the potatoes to the pan, cover with cold water and bring to the boil. Cook for 10 minutes and then add the courgette.

3 Cook for a further 5–10 minutes, until the potato feels soft.

4 Carefully drain off any excess water and mash really well using a potato masher.

5 Add a little dash of olive oil to the mash if needed.

Optional Extras
Add some dairy-free sunflower spread if desired. Also any extra chopped vegetables can be added during the cooking process – cabbage, kale and peas are all great.

PREP: 5 MINUTES
COOK: 50 MINUTES

The French call this style of cooking 'en papillote' and it is a novel way to cook and serve new potatoes. The kids always think it is really fun to be served their potatoes in a little bag at the table. Take care when opening the bags though as they are steaming hot. You can make the parcels a day in advance and pop them in the fridge until you are ready to cook.

NEW POTATOES
Cooked in a Parcel

650g baby new potatoes
Olive oil, for drizzling
A fresh rosemary sprig,
  roughly broken into
  pieces

1 Preheat the oven to 220°C/200°C fan/425°F/Gas mark 7.

2 Put the potatoes in a bowl, drizzle with olive oil and sprinkle with the rosemary. Mix together so the potatoes have a light coating of oil and herbs.

3 Place a portion of potatoes and rosemary onto a sheet of baking paper (don't be tempted to use foil as it does not work well) and wrap it up tightly so no steam can escape. You can make this in one large parcel but we prefer to make smaller, individual parcels. Place your parcels on a baking tray.

4 Bake in the oven for 50 minutes.

SERVES A FAMILY OF **4**

PREP: 5 MINUTES
COOK: 50 MINUTES

Wedges are so easy and a great alternative to chips, but with the same appeal. You can also use sweet potatoes to make a change. These wedges go well with our Lamb Kebabs (see page 118). Cammie loves these on their own with a generous squirt of ketchup for a substantial snack.

POTATO WEDGES

900g floury potatoes, such as Maris Piper, washed and left unpeeled

Sunflower or olive oil, for drizzling

1 fresh thyme sprig (optional)

Freshly ground black pepper

1 Preheat the oven to 220°C/200°C fan/425°F/Gas mark 7.

2 Slice the potatoes in half and then cut into wedges, leaving the skin on.

3 Place the wedges in a baking tray and drizzle with oil so they are very lightly coated. Season with black pepper and a sprig of thyme.

4 Bake in the oven for about 50 minutes or until the wedges are golden brown and cooked through.

If you are not allergic
Serve with a dollop of mayonnaise.

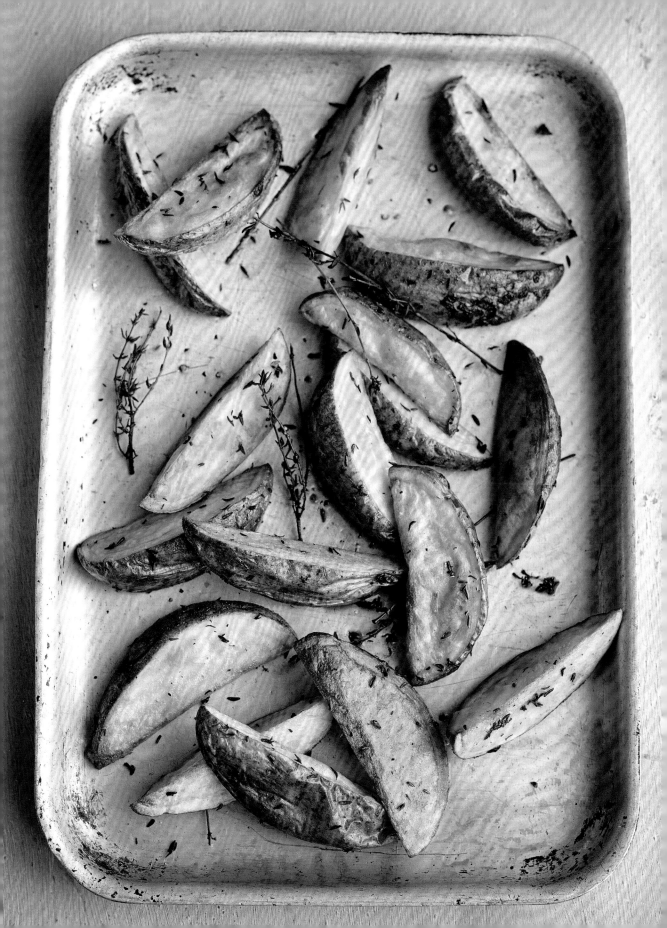

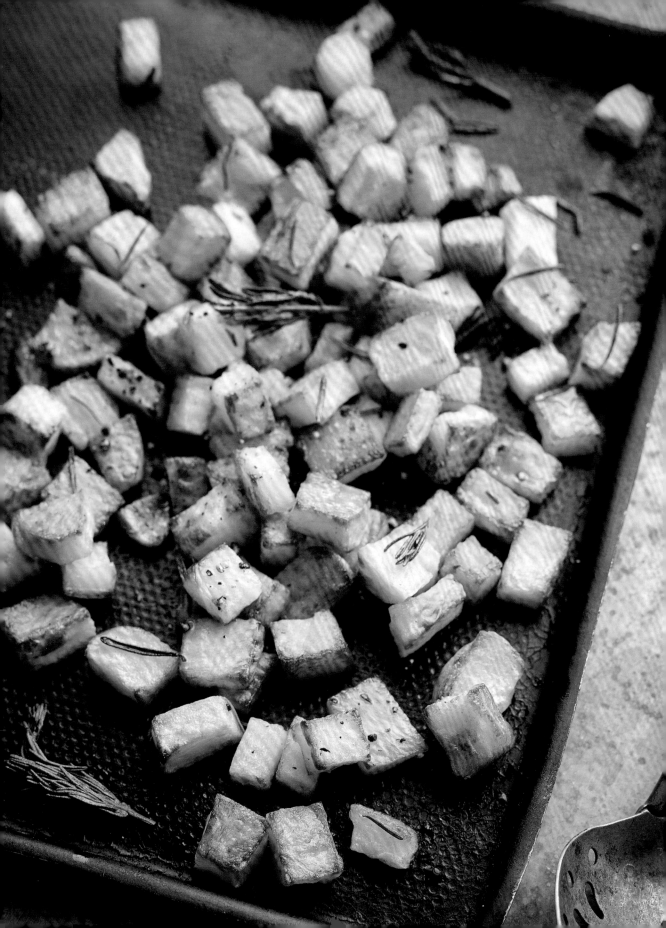

SERVES A FAMILY OF 4

PREP: 5 MINUTES
COOK: 30 MINUTES

These are small cubes or chunks of potato that are oven roasted with a little rosemary and with some added bacon, as suggested below, they are even more delicious. These are very popular with Izzy and Zara.

Parmentier POTATOES

500g floury potatoes, such as Maris Piper, peeled and chopped into small cubes
2 garlic cloves, peeled and cut in half
A fresh rosemary sprig
Sunflower oil, for drizzling

1 Preheat the oven to 220°C/200°C fan/425°F/Gas mark 7.

2 Pop the potatoes, garlic and rosemary in a baking tray and drizzle with oil.

3 Roast in the oven for about 30 minutes, shaking the tray every so often to move the potatoes around, until they are golden brown and tender in the centre.

Optional Extras
Sprinkle over 2 chopped uncooked bacon rashers before you pop the potatoes in the oven.

We think it is great to expose our kids to a range of flavours and this is a nice introduction to Indian food. It is a mild curry that is not overpowering for little ones and goes well with plain grilled chicken. It tastes best when it has been made a day in advance and then reheated.

Mild POTATO CURRY

1 tablespoon olive oil

1 small onion, sliced

1 garlic clove, crushed

1 teaspoon whole cumin seeds

¼ teaspoon ground turmeric

2 teaspoons mild curry powder (or to taste)

Small pinch salt (optional)

3 large floury potatoes, such as Maris Piper, peeled and roughly chopped

400g tin chopped tomatoes

200ml water

5 cubes (140g) supermarket frozen spinach portions or 170g fresh spinach leaves, washed

Handful fresh coriander, chopped

1 Heat the oil in a large frying pan over a medium heat and fry the onion for about 5 minutes until it softens and starts to take on a little colour.

2 Add the garlic, cumin, turmeric, curry powder and salt (if using), and stir in well.

3 Add the potatoes, tomatoes and water and gently simmer until the potatoes are tender.

4 Add the frozen or fresh spinach and cook for a further few minutes until it is all just heated through.

5 Sprinkle with coriander before serving.

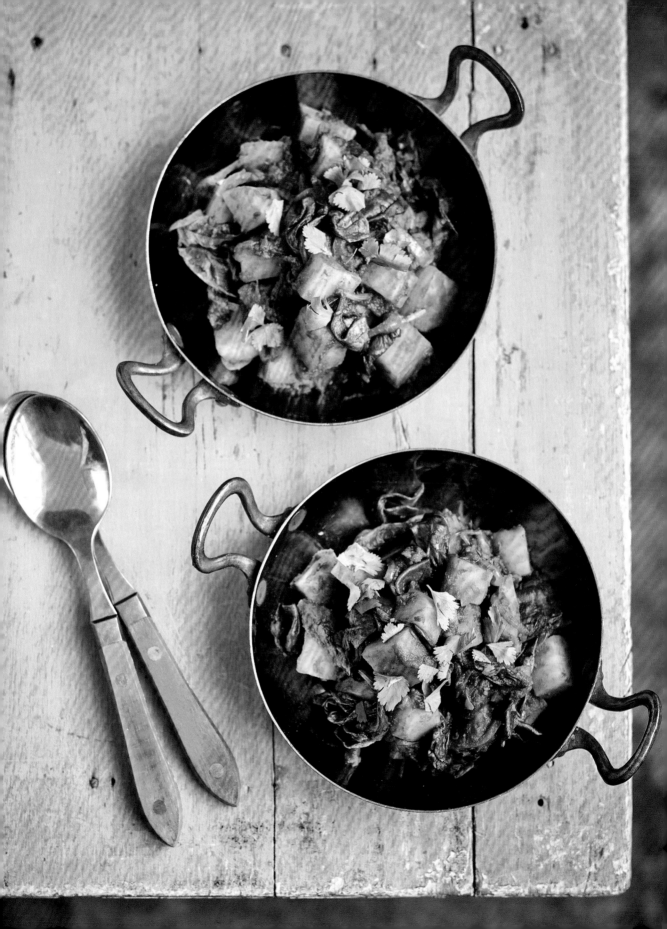

PREP: 5 MINUTES
COOK: 1 HOUR

There is no chilli in this sauce but if your kids like a little heat, you can add a pinch of chilli powder to taste. It really tastes better to make the tomato sauce a day ahead so the flavours can mellow and infuse. But if you haven't got time don't worry. Isabelle is a big fan of this dish as she really likes paprika.

Spanish PATATAS BRAVAS

650g floury potatoes, such as Maris Piper, roughly chopped
Oil, for drizzling
Small handful fresh parsley, chopped

Sauce
2 tablespoons olive oil
1 small onion, finely chopped
1 large garlic clove, crushed
400ml tomato passata
1 teaspoon sweet smoked paprika
½ teaspoon caster sugar
Freshly ground black pepper

1 First make the sauce. Heat the oil in a frying pan and gently cook the onion for a few minutes until soft. Add the garlic and cook for a further minute.

2 Add the rest of the sauce ingredients and cook for a further 10 minutes. If your kids prefer a completely smooth sauce just blitz it quickly with a handheld blender.

3 Leave the sauce to cool and then pop in the fridge overnight.

4 Preheat the oven to 220°C/200°C fan/425°F/ Gas mark 7.

5 Put the potatoes in a roasting tin and drizzle with a little oil. Bake in the oven for about 50 minutes until cooked.

6 Reheat the sauce in a saucepan. Pour the sauce over the potatoes once cooked and then sprinkle with parsley before serving.

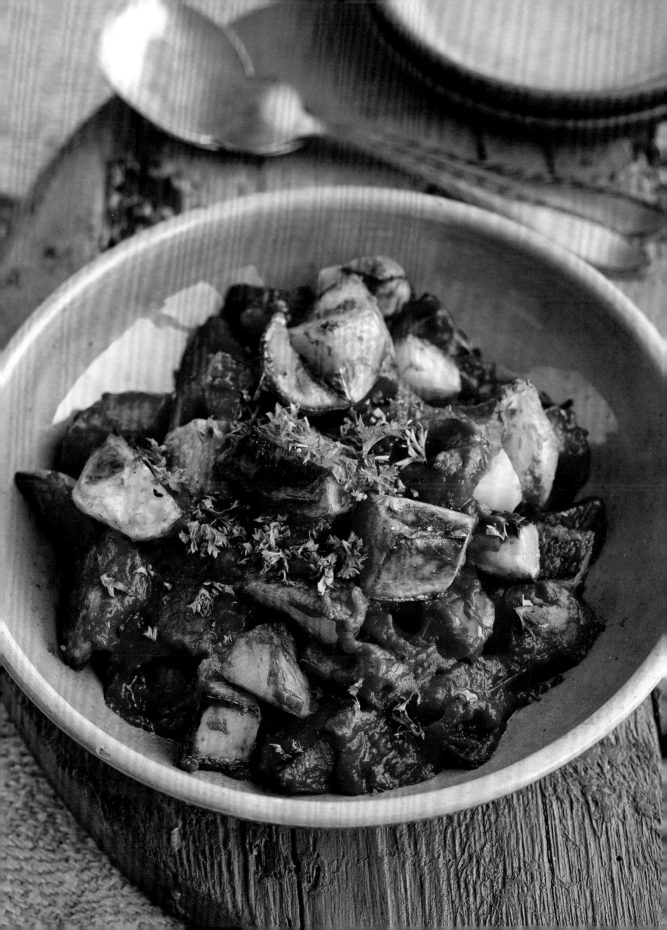

With delicious crispy skin and beautifully fluffy potato on the inside, jacket potatoes are an easy meal and great with a variety of different toppings. Cook an extra potato to chill overnight and have for breakfast the next day, just chopped up and heated through. If you are short on time, microwave the potato for a while before placing it in the oven, although this may mean the skin is not as crispy.

SERVES
A FAMILY OF
4

PREP: 5 MINUTES
COOK: 1½ HOURS

Jacket POTATOES

4 baking potatoes, washed (most supermarkets sell 'baking' potatoes or Roosters are good)

Other Topping Suggestions

- Dairy-free sunflower spread
- Three Bean Salad (see page 142)
- Sweetcorn
- Chilli con Carne (See page 54)
- Ratatouille (see page 166)
- Baked beans
- Tinned fish
… just to name a few.

1 Preheat the oven to 220°C/200°C fan/425°F/Gas mark 7.

2 Stick a fork in the side of the whole unpeeled potatoes – this will help prevent them exploding in the oven.

3 Place the potatoes directly onto the middle shelf in the oven, and cook for about 1–1½ hours.

4 Cut the potatoes in half and fill with your chosen topping, taking care as the potatoes will be very hot.

If you are not allergic
Serve with butter and grated cheese.

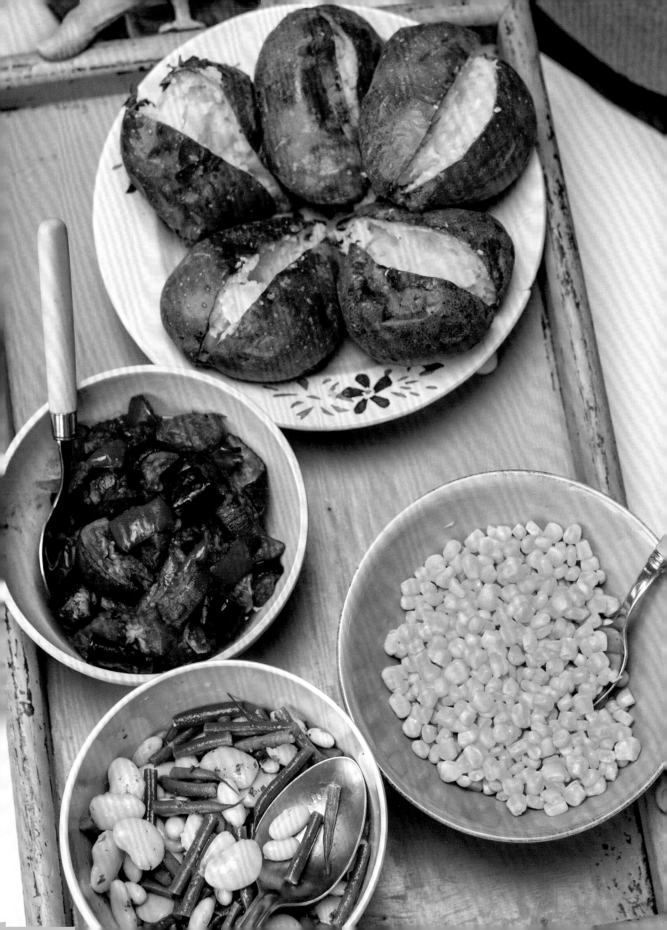

This is a simple way to enhance plain boiled rice and is really nice with any Thai or Indian dishes, such as Mild Thai Coconut Chicken Curry (see page 48) or Mild Fish Curry (see page 102). This recipe calls for creamed coconut – not the coconut cream or milk that you find in tins but in little packets containing small sachets. These contain desiccated coconut and need to be mixed in boiling water before using. They are easy to find in supermarkets, are very simple to use and produce a lovely flavour.

SERVES
A FAMILY OF
4

PREP: 5 MINUTES
COOK: 20 MINUTES

Coconut RICE

½ teaspoon olive oil
¼ cinnamon stick
¼ small onion, finely chopped
2 garlic cloves, crushed
Handful fresh coriander leaves, finely chopped, plus ½ teaspoon chopped stems
200g white rice (either Thai jasmine or basmati)
50g sachet creamed coconut mixed in 400ml boiling water
1 lime, to serve

1 Heat the oil in a heavy-based pan over a medium heat and add the cinnamon stick, onion, garlic and chopped coriander stems and fry for a couple of minutes until the onion starts to soften.

2 Add the rice and stir through and then add the creamed coconut. Cover with a lid and simmer over a low heat for 10 minutes.

3 Remove the pan from the heat, leaving the lid on and rest for a further 5 minutes. All the liquid should have been absorbed into the rice and the rice should be tender.

4 Remove the cinnamon stick and discard. Fluff the rice up with a fork and add a good squeeze of lime juice and the chopped coriander leaves. Serve immediately.

> *If you are not allergic*
> 60g unsalted cashew nuts can be added at the very first stage with the cinnamon, onion and garlic.

PREP: 5 MINUTES
COOK: 15 MINUTES

This is a quick and easy meal or side dish. For convenience you can use prepared stir-fry vegetable bags from the supermarket or whatever vegetables you have handy at home instead of the vegetables we suggest. If you choose to use brown rice, the cooking time will be longer.

Stir-Fried RICE

250g long-grain rice
2 teaspoons sunflower oil
½ red onion, finely sliced
6 green cabbage leaves, finely sliced
1 large carrot, peeled and then sliced into ribbons using a vegetable peeler
Good handful of beansprouts
Small pinch Chinese five-spice (optional) !

1 Boil the rice in a saucepan of water according to the packet instructions – it normally takes 12 minutes for white rice and 30 minutes for brown rice. Drain well once cooked.

2 Heat the oil in a large frying pan or wok over medium heat and stir fry the onion for a few minutes until softened.

3 Add the cabbage and carrot and stir fry for a couple more minutes. Finally add the beansprouts and Chinese five-spice, if using, and keep mixing well.

4 Add the rice and keep moving in the pan for a minute to heat through and then serve immediately.

If you are not allergic

Make egg-fried rice by cracking an egg into a bowl and whisking well. Add this to the pan at step 4 with the rice and stir furiously so that the egg disperses and cooks in with the rice.

Note
Some Chinese five-spice seasoning packets have a whole range of added ingredients such as salt and sugar as well as allergens. Make sure yours contains just cinnamon, fennel, star anise, ginger and cloves.

SERVES A FAMILY OF 4

PREP: 5 MINUTES
COOK: 15 MINUTES

This is a lovely rice to serve with our Ever-so-Mild Chicken Korma (see page 110) or Moroccan Spiced Lamb Tagine (see page 60). It really doesn't take much longer than plain boiled rice and the results are much tastier.

PILAU RICE
with Fruit

2 teaspoons olive oil
½ onion, finely sliced
1 teaspoon whole
    cumin seeds
2 cardamom pods
1 teaspoon whole
    coriander seeds
280g white basmati rice
550ml water
½ cinnamon stick
15g raisins
20g dried apricots,
    finely chopped
Freshly ground black
    pepper

1 Heat the oil in a heavy-based pan over a medium heat and fry the onion, cumin, cardamom and coriander until the onion is soft and a little brown.

2 Add the rice, water and cinnamon, bring to the boil, then turn down the heat, cover with a lid and simmer gently for 10 minutes.

3 Check if the rice is tender and all the water absorbed. It may need a few more minutes of cooking if this is not the case.

4 Remove the cinnamon stick and cardamom pods.

5 Stir in the raisins, apricots, black pepper and rest for a further minute.

6 Fluff with a fork and serve.

If you are not allergic

Add about 40g of any tree nuts that you like at the end of the cooking process – unsalted pistachios, almonds and cashews are all great with this. Also, lots of other dried fruit work well, such as currants, prunes and dried figs, as long as you use small pieces.

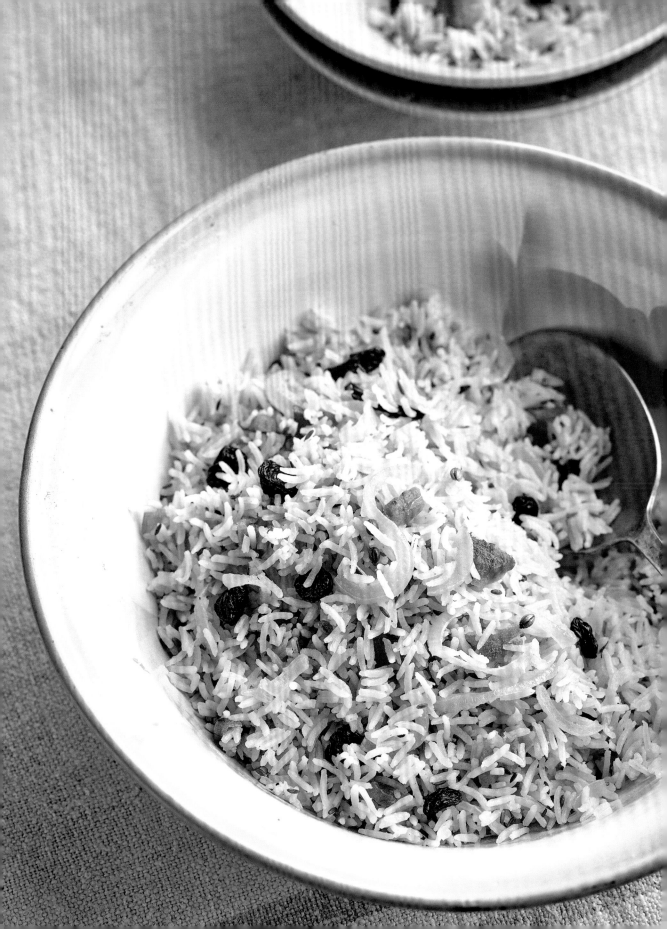

MAKES
12
PIECES

PREP: 25 MINUTES
COOK: 15 MINUTES

Sushi is Casper's absolute favourite for packed lunches, picnics or anytime really. It might sound a bit daunting to make your own sushi but give it a go – it is really easy and it's great fun to get the kids involved in making their own too. This is such a good portable meal for those who cannot eat gluten. Most supermarkets will sell little bamboo mats that you can use to help you roll up the sushi, but a clean tea towel will also work.

Avocado MAKI SUSHI

120g sushi rice
200ml water
1 teaspoon mirin
2 teaspoons Japanese
   rice vinegar
2 sheets sushi nori
3 thin slices of avocado

If you are not allergic

This is great with a little soy sauce or tamari if you need to use a wheat-free soya sauce.

Other Filling Suggestions

· cucumber sliced into sticks
· smoked salmon cut into
   slithers
· smoked mackerel flaked
   into slices
· red pepper cut into slices
· yellow pepper cut
   into slices
· grated carrot
· chives bundled together
· shredded chicken
· shredded duck

1 Rinse the sushi rice under the tap and place in a small saucepan. Add the water and leave to soak for 30 minutes (if you don't have time just move on to the next stage).

2 Put a lid on the pan and bring to the boil. As soon as it boils, turn down to a very gentle simmer for 10 minutes or until the rice is cooked – don't lift the lid too much as the steam cooks the rice and you don't want it all to escape.

3 Mix the vinegar and mirin in a small cup.

4 When the rice has cooked, tip it out onto a plate and pour over the vinegar and mirin. Move the rice around the plate with a spatula until the rice has cooled to room temperature – you can fan the rice with a magazine or plastic plate to help speed up the process.

5 Lay a sheet of nori, shiny side down, on a sushi mat or clean tea towel covered with some clingfilm, and spread a layer of rice over two-thirds of the nori.

6 Add strips of avocado, or whatever filling you like, in the centre of the rice, in a line and then roll into a sausage shape using the sushi mat or tea towel to help get an even roll.

7 Repeat for the second piece of nori.

8 Cut each roll into 6 pieces using a sharp knife.

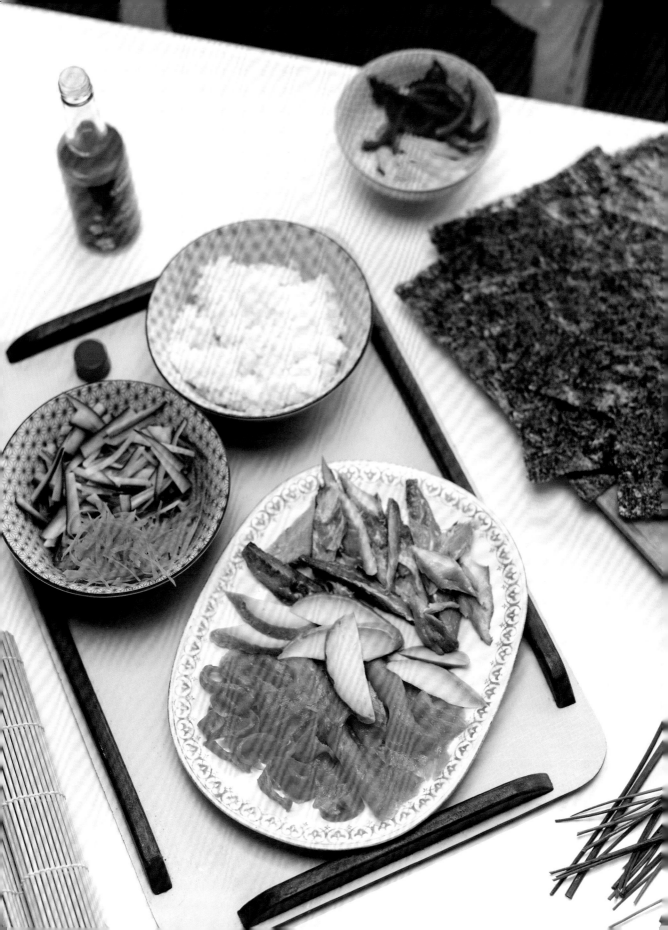

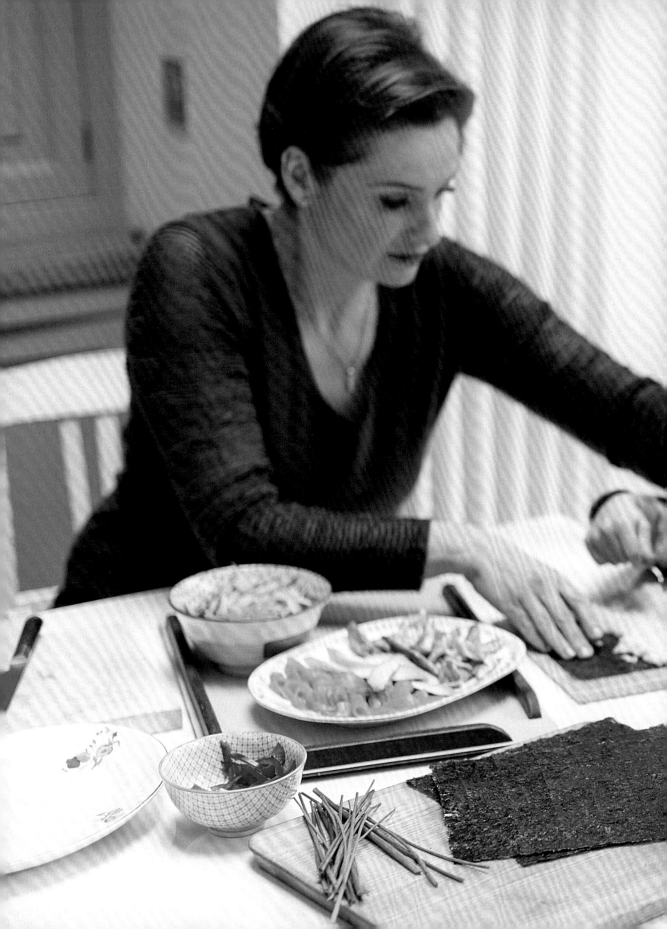

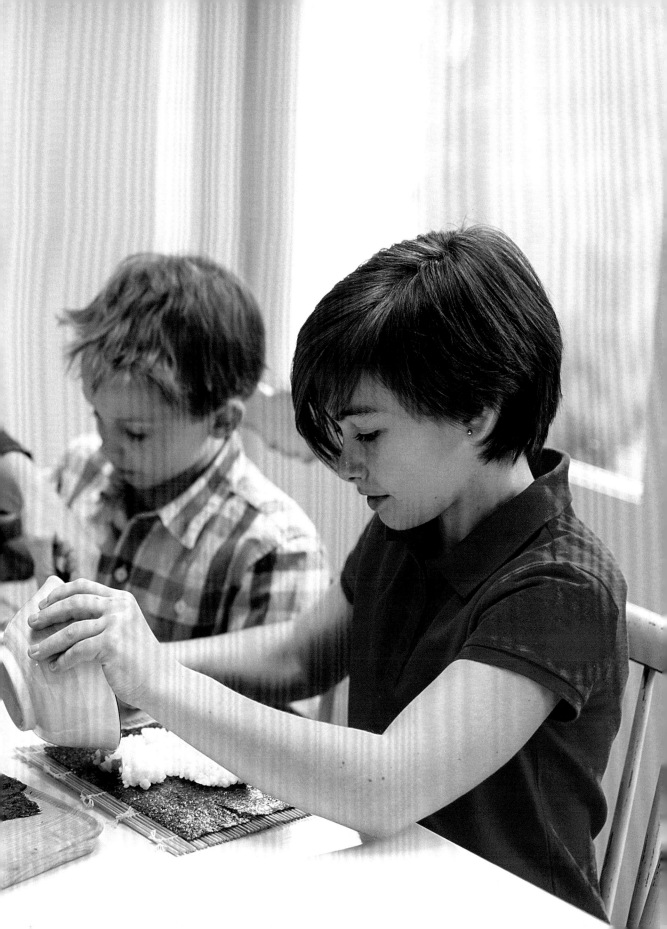

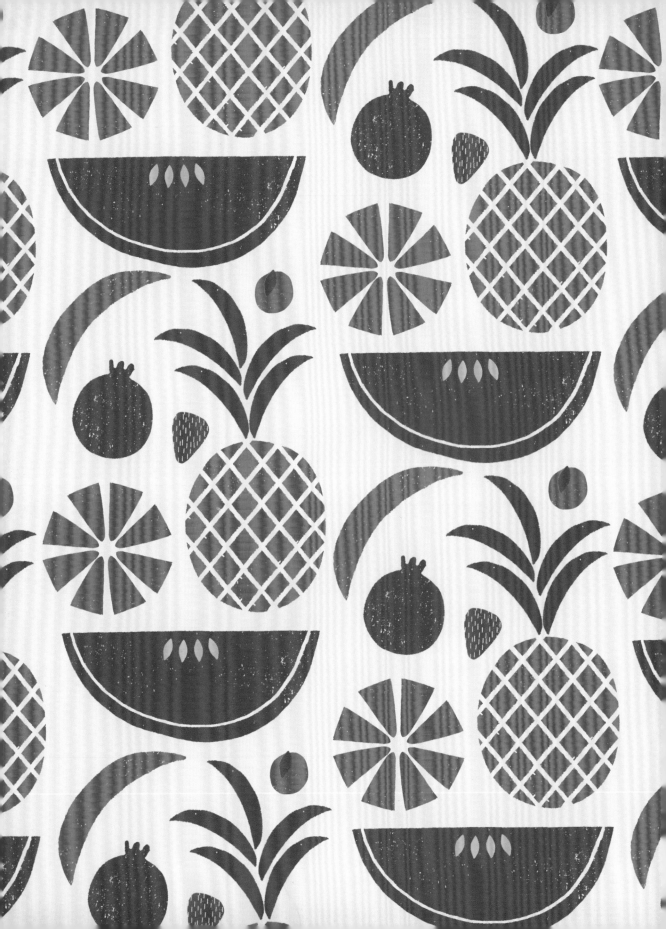

Sweet Things

There's no better dessert than a piece of fresh fruit and it's an easy way of contributing to the five portions of fruit and vegetables we should all have every day. However, when you want to give your children a treat there are great free-from ice creams and cornets and a few completely free-from puddings available in most supermarkets. If your children can have dairy, soya or egg then they will have a large choice of ready-made yoghurts and desserts, just remember to check the labels carefully.

When you have a bit more time you can try some of our recipes for cakes and sweet things that are completely free from the eight most common allergens.

NOTES ON BAKING

Baking and making cakes with no dairy, eggs or gluten can be a challenge.

When making a totally free-from cake we recommend that you use a set of measuring spoons and electronic scales so your quantities are accurate and you get the best results.

Some of our recipes call for xanthum gum, which is readily available in most supermarkets where there are several brands to choose from. It helps bind the ingredients, which is crucial in the absence of egg or gluten.

All kids love chocolate and if your child has a dairy allergy there is no need to miss out; there are lots of options. In the shops there are typically dairy-free and soya lecithin-free brands; there are brands that make dark chocolate without dairy in factories that are totally safe from nuts, but contain soy lecithin; and other easy-to-obtain dark chocolate brands that are free from all allergens in their ingredients but may contain traces of allergens due to the factory they are processed in.

In the recipes where we use chocolate, please use a brand that you are comfortable with. All the recipes work well with both dairy-free chocolate and dark chocolate that is naturally dairy free.

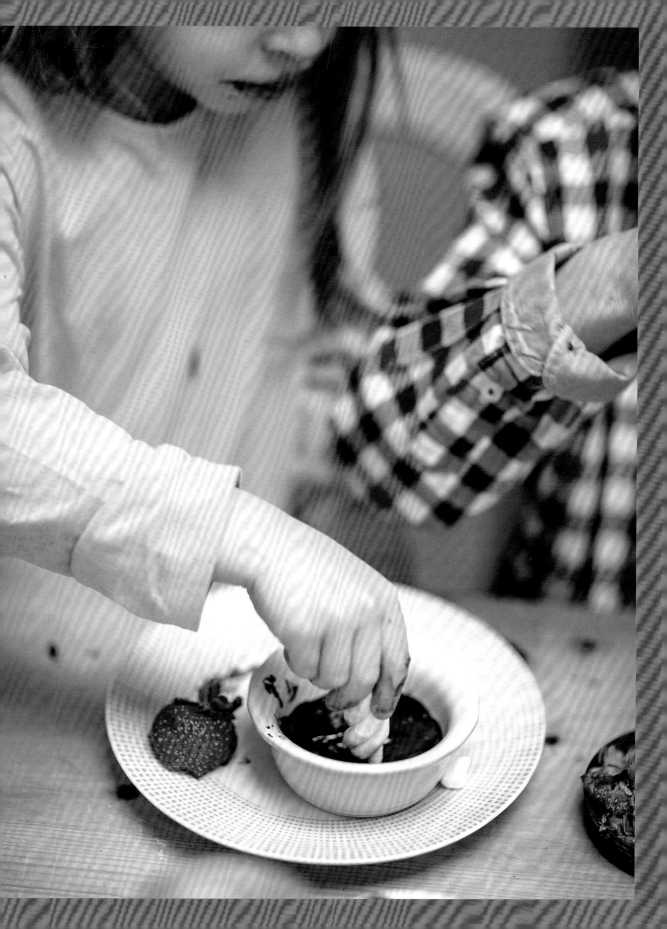

FRUIT SMOOTHIES

SERVES 2 CHILDREN

PREP: 5 MINUTES
COOK: NONE

Smoothies can be a quick and easy breakfast option when you're pressed for time and they are also a good way of eating more fruit. You can measure the ingredients out carefully or just use the glass you are going to drink out of, pile it in and then tip into the blender.

The Pink One

2 good handfuls seedless
   white grapes (about 20)
½ banana
2 good handfuls frozen
   raspberries (about 30)
125ml pineapple juice
125ml coconut cream
   (optional)

This is really just a raspberry smoothie but our kids request their smoothies by colour and so this is the Pink One.

Put all the ingredients in a blender and blitz until smooth.

The White One

100ml coconut cream
   from a tin or carton
½ banana (about 50g)
125ml pineapple juice
   from a carton

A delicious coconut and banana smoothie using fruit you have in your fruit bowl at home and juice from cartons in the fridge.

Put all the ingredients in a blender and blitz until smooth. Serve with a few ice cubes.

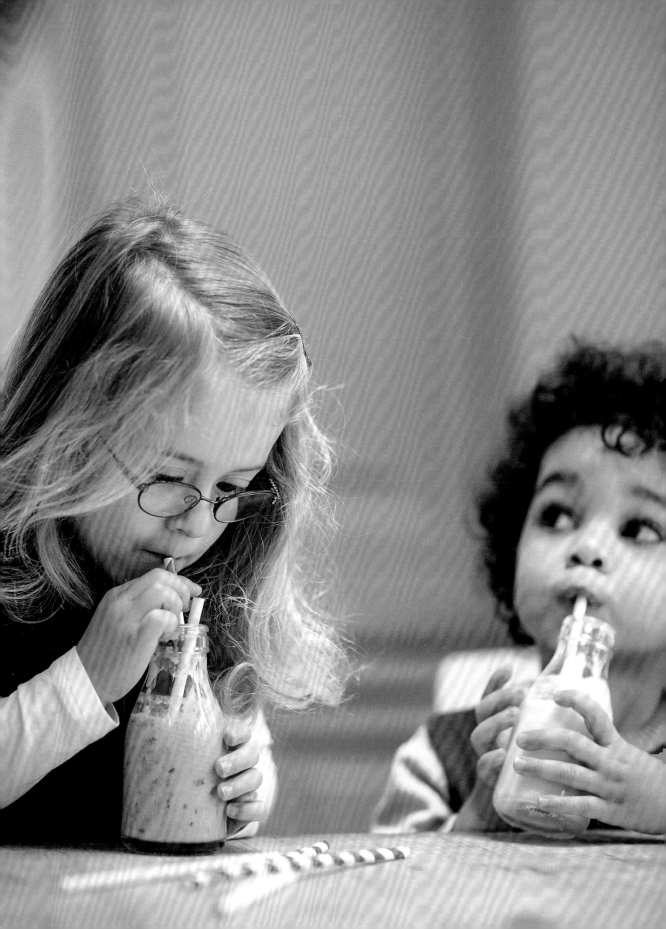

SERVES A FAMILY OF 4

PREP: 15 MINUTES
COOK: 35 MINUTES

If you have any bananas getting too ripe in your fruit bowl this is the perfect way to use them up – the riper the better! This is best served freshly made with some dairy-free sunflower spread or if you want to be a bit more fancy it is yummy with a little lemon drizzle icing on top. Remember that raising agents only start to work when they come into contact with moisture so as soon as you combine the wet and dry ingredients, work quickly and put your mixture in the oven as soon as you can.

BANANA BREAD

3 large, over-ripe bananas (about 350g)
60g caster sugar
55ml vegetable oil
1 tablespoon fresh lemon juice
1 tablespoon rice milk
210g gluten-free self-raising flour
1 teaspoon gluten-free baking powder
½ teaspoon bicarbonate of soda
¼ teaspoon xantham gum
⅛ teaspoon salt

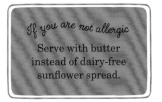

If you are not allergic
Serve with butter instead of dairy-free sunflower spread.

1 Preheat the oven to 200°C/190°C fan/400°F/Gas mark 6. Line a 500g/1lb loaf tin with baking paper.

2 Use a stand mixer, or mix by hand, to combine the bananas with the sugar, vegetable oil, lemon juice and milk in a bowl.

3 Thoroughly mix the flour, baking powder, bicarbonate of soda, xantham gum and salt in a separate bowl.

4 Tip the dry ingredients into the banana mixture and mix well either by hand or with a stand mixer.

5 Don't hang around – as soon as the mixture is combined pour into the prepared tin. Tap the tin on your work surface to remove any large air bubbles and place on the middle shelf in your oven immediately.

6 Bake for about 30–35 minutes (test with a skewer or sharp knife – if it comes out clean without any raw mixture, it is cooked). Leave to cool in the tin for 5 minutes before turning onto a wire rack to cool.

7 Slice and serve with a topping of dairy-free sunflower spread.

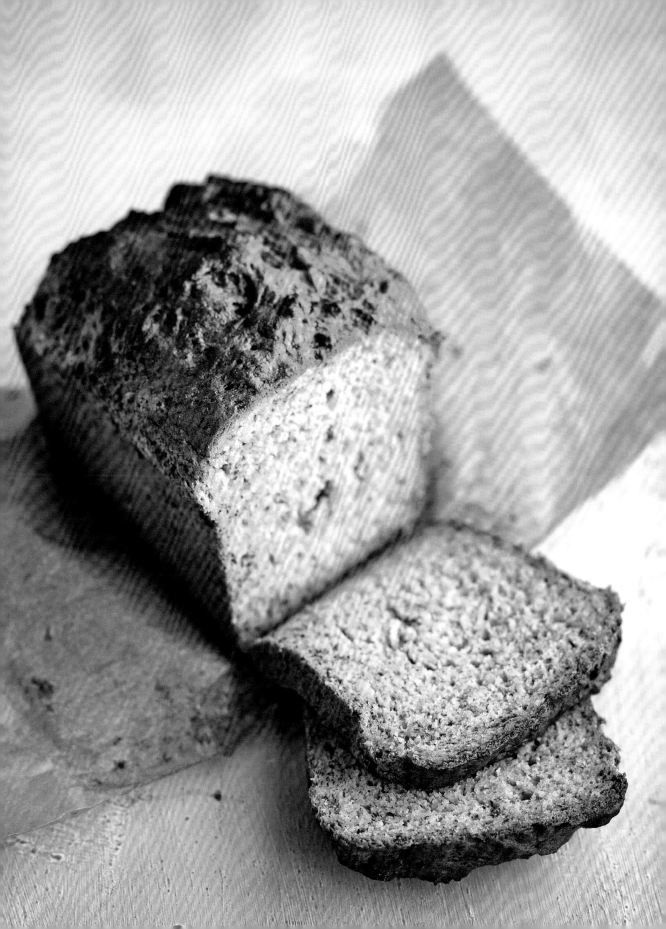

SERVES 8-12

PREP: 15 MINUTES
COOK: 35 MINUTES

This cake is great for a birthday or celebration and is a huge hit with everyone who eats it. You can also use this mixture to make 12 large cupcakes or 24 little ones, but remember to reduce the cooking time to 15–20 minutes. You can easily freeze these complete with icing and defrost an hour or so before they are needed.

Really Chocolatey CHOCOLATE CAKE

450ml rice milk
1 tablespoon cider vinegar
300g caster sugar
300g gluten-free self-raising flour, sifted
100g cocoa powder, sifted
1 tablespoon gluten-free baking powder
1 teaspoon bicarbonate of soda
¼ teaspoon xantham gum
Pinch salt
160ml sunflower oil
2 tablespoons vanilla extract

Icing
225g dairy-free sunflower spread
225g icing sugar, sifted
50g cocoa powder, sifted
100g dairy-free dark chocolate (70% cocoa)

To decorate
Dairy-free chocolate buttons
or fresh berries

1 Preheat the oven to 220°C/200°C fan/425°F/Gas mark 7. Line the base of two 20cm cake tins with baking paper and lightly grease the paper and tins with oil.

2 Mix the rice milk and cider vinegar together and set aside. Don't worry if it separates – you are effectively making a buttermilk that will give the cake a light texture and help to activate the raising agents.

3 Mix the sugar, flour, cocoa powder, baking powder, bicarb of soda, xantham gum and salt together in a bowl. Make sure they are really well mixed together.

4 Pour the oil, vanilla and the rice milk and vinegar mixture into the dry ingredients. Mix them together really well either by hand or gently using an handheld blender.

5 Divide the mixture between the two prepared tins. Tap the tins on your work surface to remove any large air bubbles and place on the middle shelf in the oven. Bake for about 30–35 minutes (test with a skewer or sharp knife – if it comes out clean it is cooked).

6 Leave the cakes to cool in their tins for 5 minutes before turning out onto wire racks to cool completely.

7 To make the icing, whisk the sunflower spread, icing sugar and cocoa powder in a bowl. Break the chocolate up into pieces in a microwave-safe bowl and cook on high in 10-second bursts until it has just melted. Add the melted chocolate to the icing and mix.

8 Spread an even layer of icing on one of the cooled cakes and then place the other cake on top. Top the cake with the rest of the icing. Decorate with dairy-free chocolate buttons (or fresh berries if preferred).

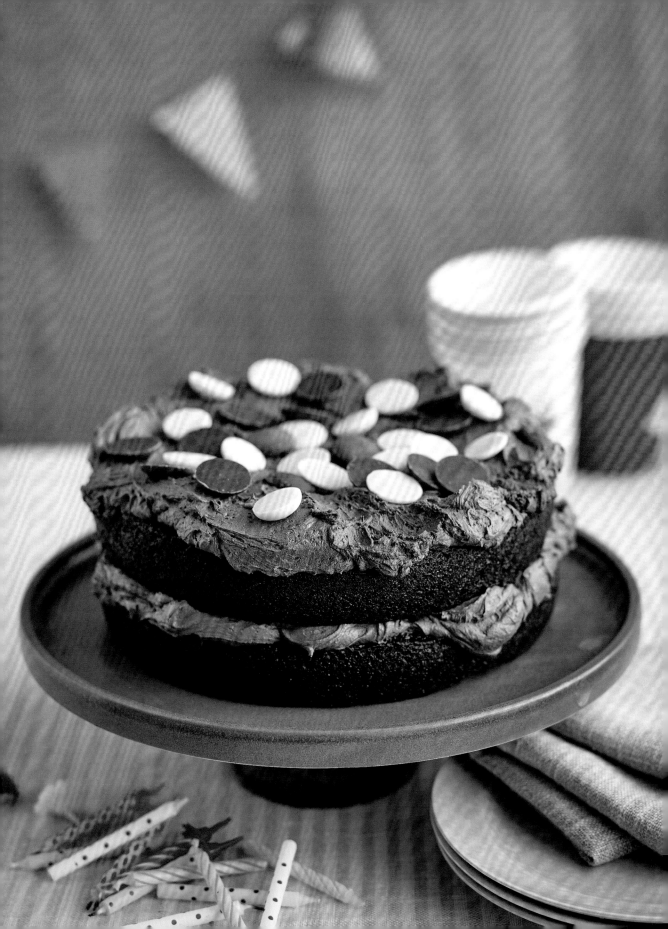

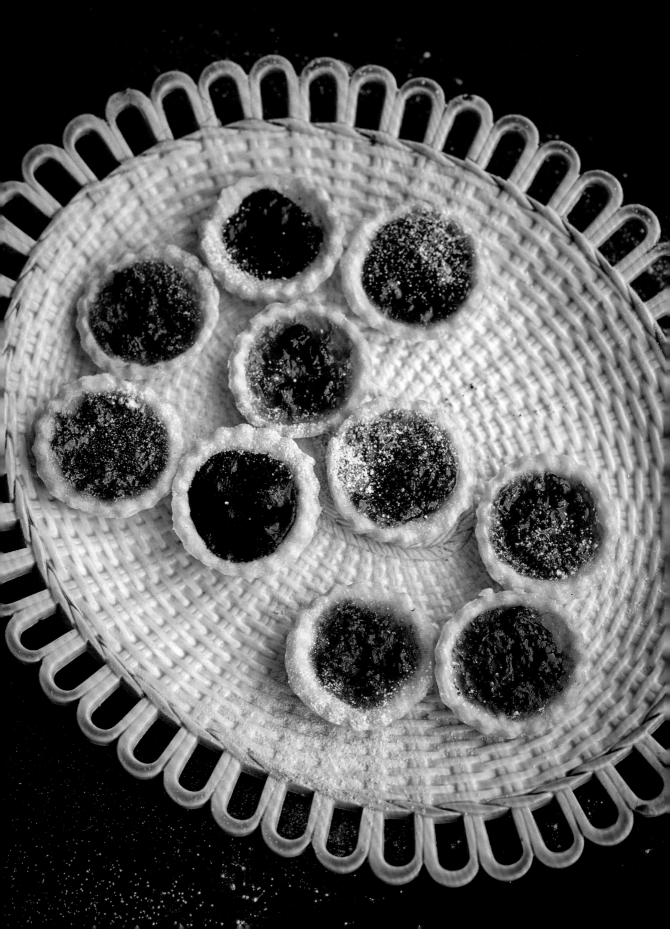

PREP: 15 MINUTES, PLUS CHILLING COOK: 15 MINUTES

Children love making jam tarts. This pastry recipe makes quite a crisp, biscuity pastry that is really delicious; it is not soft like the ready-made pastry you get with manufactured jam tarts or mince pies. Making pastry is very easy and takes moments – remember to keep the ingredients cool for success every time. It is vital that the dairy-free sunflower spread is very cold or the recipe will not work – you can always pop it in the freezer for a while if it is too soft.

Jam TARTS

170g gluten-free flour, plus extra for dusting
85g dairy-free sunflower spread
2 tablespoons caster sugar
Jam, to fill (any flavour you like!)

If you are not allergic

Use butter instead of dairy-free sunflower spread. If your child can eat wheat flour, use this instead of gluten-free flour.

Christmas Mince Pies

At Christmas time simply fill your pastry cases with mincemeat. **!** Using a 5cm fluted cutter, make a pastry lid to place on top. Out of the lid you can cut little star or holly shapes to make them look extra pretty and this way you can see the mincemeat through the hole. Alternatively, put a pastry star on top.

---

1 Place the flour and spread in a blender or food processor and pulse quickly until it looks like breadcrumbs.

2 Tip the mixture into a bowl and stir in the sugar. Add a teaspoon of cold water and begin bringing the dough together with your hands into a ball. You will probably need between 1 teaspoon and 1 tablespoon of cold water to bring it together well. It should not be sticky. Add as little water as possible to give a short texture.

3 Roll the dough out on a flat surface dusted with gluten-free flour, and cut into circles using a fluted 6cm cutter.

4 Lift the pastry discs up carefully with a slice and place them into a muffin tray, gently pushing down with your fingers. Pop them in the fridge to chill for 30 minutes. Preheat the oven to 220°C/200°C fan/ 425°F/Gas mark 7.

5 Bake the tart cases in the oven for about 10 minutes until very lightly golden and sandy in texture.

6 Spoon a generous teaspoon of your favourite jam to fill the pastry case and pop back in the oven for a few minutes until the jam starts to gently bubble.

7 Remove the tray from the oven and transfer the tarts to a wire rack, allowing them to cool fully before serving.

**PREP: 15 MINUTES,
PLUS CHILLING
COOK: 30 MINUTES**

Our kids love these small tarts that they call mud pies. One large tart that can be sliced and shared when entertaining family and friends also works well. Whichever way you make this dessert, it's quick, easy and rich with a delicious crisp, biscuity pastry. Making pastry is very easy – remember to keep the dairy-free sunflower spread very cold for perfect results.

Chocolate TARTS

170g gluten-free flour
85g dairy-free
    sunflower spread
2 tablespoons caster sugar

Filling
200g dark chocolate
    or dairy-free
    chocolate ❗
160ml tin or carton of
    coconut cream
2–3 tablespoons golden
    syrup (adjust according
    to how sweet you like it)
½ teaspoon vanilla extract

If you are not allergic
Use butter instead of dairy-free sunflower spread and use wheat flour instead of gluten-free flour. If you want to make the tart a bit more fun, add a good sprinkle of popping candy to the mixture after the vanilla has been mixed in.

1 Place the flour and spread in a blender or food processor and pulse quickly until it looks like breadcrumbs.

2 Tip the mixture into a bowl and stir in the sugar. Add a teaspoon of cold water and begin bringing the dough together with your hands into a ball. You will probably need between 1 teaspoon and 1 tablespoon of cold water to bring it together well. It should not be sticky. Add as little water as possible for a short texture.

3 Roll the dough out on a flat surface dusted with gluten-free flour and cut into circles. Carefully lift into flan rings. It helps to use a cake slice to pick up the pastry and put it into a ring, gently pushing down with your fingers. Pop the pastry into the fridge to chill for 30 minutes. Preheat the oven to 220°C/ 200°C fan/425°F/Gas mark 7.

4 Bake in the oven for 20 minutes until very lightly golden and sandy in texture. Leave to cool on a wire rack while you make your filling.

5 Put all the filling ingredients, except the vanilla, in a microwavable bowl and heat on high for 10 seconds at a time, stirring well between each go, until all the chocolate has melted and it is lovely and smooth.

6 Add in the vanilla, stir well and then pour into your pastry cases. Pop the tarts in the fridge to set for an hour or so before serving.

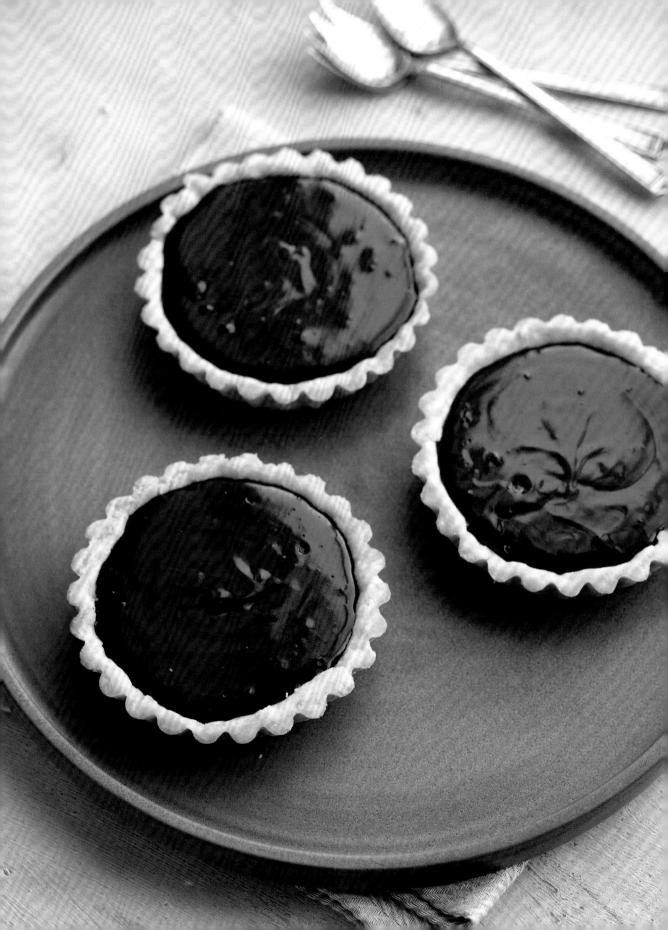

This is an old-fashioned pudding – there really is something lovely and comforting about baked apples. These are delicious on their own or with a scoop of your favourite brand of dairy-free ice cream.

Traditional BAKED APPLES

4 Bramley cooking apples
2 tablespoons raisins
2 tablespoons dried apricots, chopped
2 tablespoons dried soft dates with stone removed, chopped
50g dairy-free sunflower spread
2 tablespoons light or dark soft brown sugar

If you are not allergic
Use butter instead of sunflower spread and serve with ice cream or double cream.

1 Preheat the oven to 200°C/190°C fan/400°F/Gas mark 6.

2 Remove the core from the apples, being careful not to go all the way through to the bottom. If you don't have an apple corer you can use a sharp knife to cut around the core and then use a spoon to scoop it out.

3 Use a sharp knife to gently score around the 'equator' of the apple. This will stop the skin exploding during the cooking process.

4 Combine the dried fruit, spread and sugar in a bowl and then generously fill the cavity of the apple where the core has been removed.

5 Place the apples on a baking tray and bake in the oven for 30 minutes until lovely and soft.

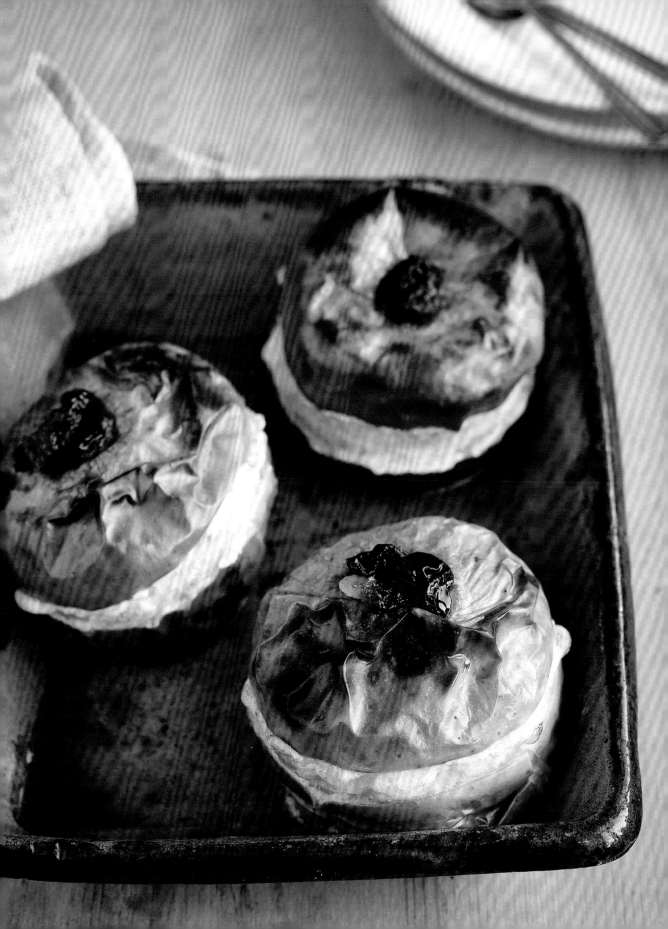

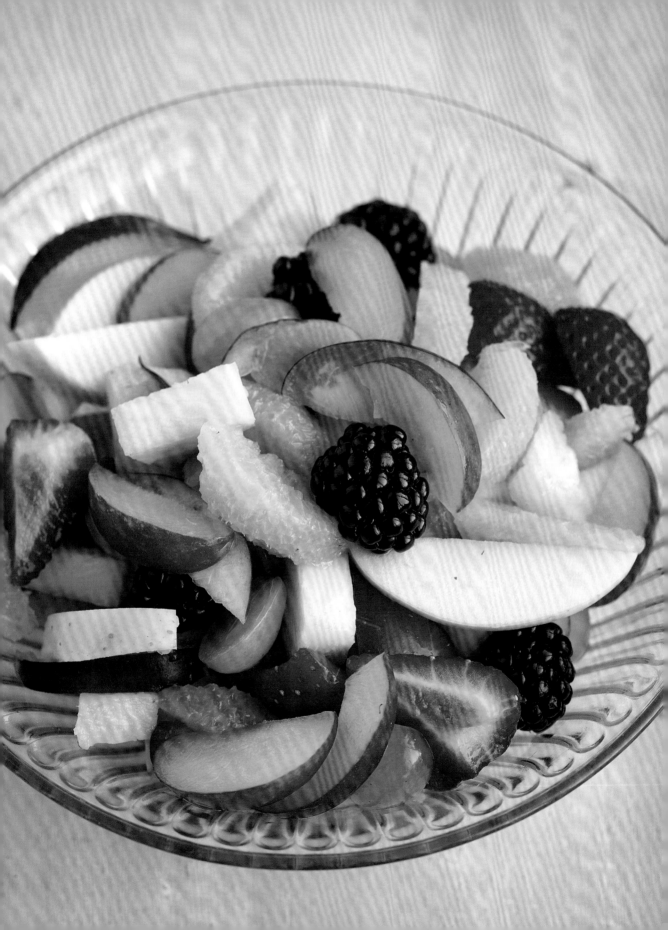

Fruit salad is easy to make; just chop up your favourite fruit and serve with a little fruit juice poured over. We have given a recipe below but you can easily add whatever fruit you happen to have at home. To make it more fun you can make serving dishes out of the fruit that you have just used, such as hollowed out melons, pineapples and grapefruits. Or if you want to go a step further, sliced fruit can also be layered up to look like a cake – use more robust fruit like melon at the bottom and more delicate berries at the top. Use the ring of a cake tin to help you keep the shape while you are layering up the fruit.

SERVES A FAMILY OF

4

PREP: 15 MINUTES
COOK: NONE

Summer
FRUIT SALAD

¼ small pineapple,
   peeled and sliced
Good handful of
   strawberries, hulled
   and cut in half
   or quartered
1 large orange,
   segmented
1 yellow nectarine,
   stoned and sliced
1 plum, stoned and sliced
Good handful of seedless
   white grapes, cut
   in half
1 green apple, sliced
Handful of blackberries
100ml freshly squeezed
   orange juice

Combine all the ingredients in a serving bowl and top with the fruit juice.

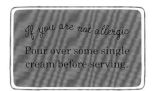

If you are not allergic
Pour over some single cream before serving.

The longer the pears sit in this citrusy syrup the better they will taste. These are delicious eaten as soon as they are cooked but they can be prepared in advance and kept in the fridge in their syrup, for up to two days to let the flavours develop. Any excess syrup can also be stored in the fridge for a few days and is lovely drizzled on vanilla dairy-free ice cream.

Poached PEARS

225g caster sugar
350ml water
Peel of 1 unwaxed lemon
Juice of 1 lemon
1 cinnamon stick
1 teaspoon vanilla
   extract
4 pears

1 Select a saucepan that fits 4 pears snugly and add the sugar and water. Warm over a low heat until the sugar has dissolved.

2 Take the pan off the heat and add the lemon peel, lemon juice, cinnamon and vanilla.

3 Peel the pears carefully to ensure all the skin is removed and place them in the saucepan of syrup as soon as they are peeled to stop them going brown.

4 Once all the pears are peeled and in the pan, place it back over a low heat and return it to a simmer. Turn the pears occasionally if they are not totally covered in the liquid (this will depend on your size of pan).

5 Simmer for about 20 minutes or until the pears are soft. Leave to cool in the syrup for a few moments before serving. Alternatively, they are just as good eaten cold.

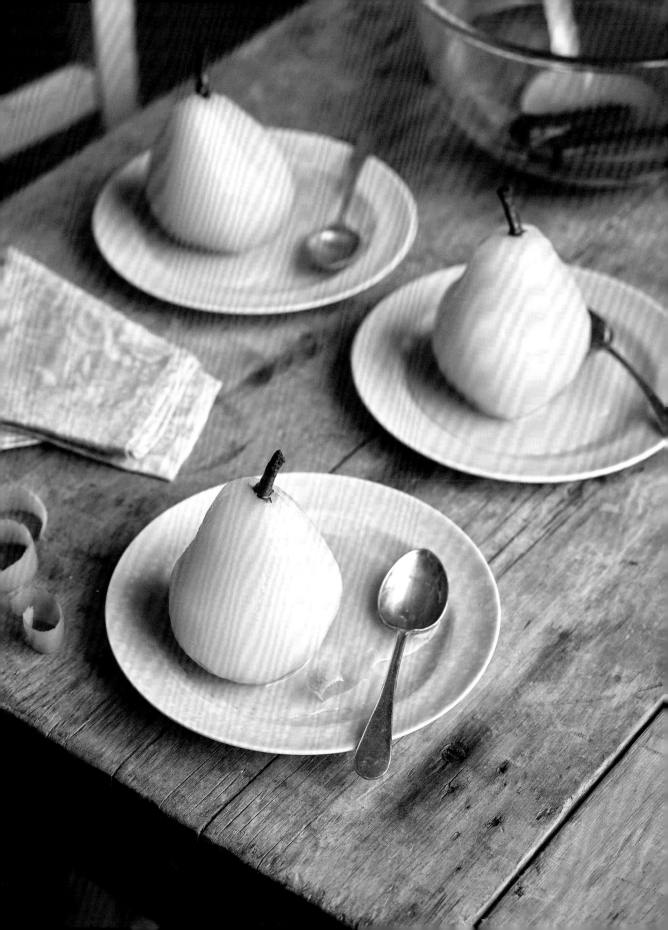

PREP: 5 MINUTES
COOK: 10 MINUTES

This is an impressive pudding that is very quick and easy. We find having a bag of frozen berries in the freezer is really handy for this recipe and also for smoothies (see page 206). This sauce also works really well with segments of orange. Most supermarkets sell bags of frozen berries individually or as mixes, which are ideal for this recipe. Avoid large fruit as it will take too long to defrost – small berries are best.

BERRIES
with Caramel Sauce

Good handful of
  frozen raspberries
  and blackcurrants
  (or whatever frozen
  berry mix you have
  in the freezer)
50g granulated sugar
100ml water
90ml orange juice

1 Spread out a good handful of frozen berries in 4 serving bowls and leave them to defrost just a little while you make the sauce.

2 Put the sugar and water in a heavy-based pan and slowly heat until the sugar has dissolved. Once it has dissolved avoid stirring as this can interfere with the sugar turning into a nice caramel and can cause it to crystallise.

3 Increase the heat and let the caramel boil for about 4½ minutes until it turns a nice deep caramel colour. Watch carefully as the caramel can turn quickly from perfect to burned.

4 Remove from the heat and add the orange juice but be careful as it will bubble furiously.

5 Stir well, returning to the heat again if needed to bring the sauce back to a runny consistency.

6 Pour the hot sauce over the fruit. The hot sauce will defrost the fruit so let it sit for a few moments before you enjoy it.

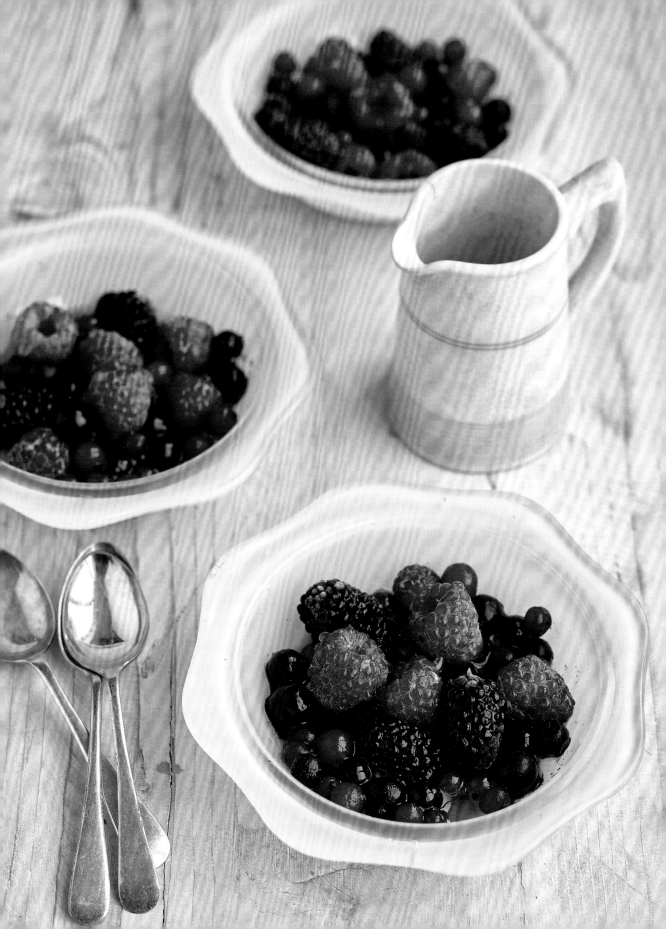

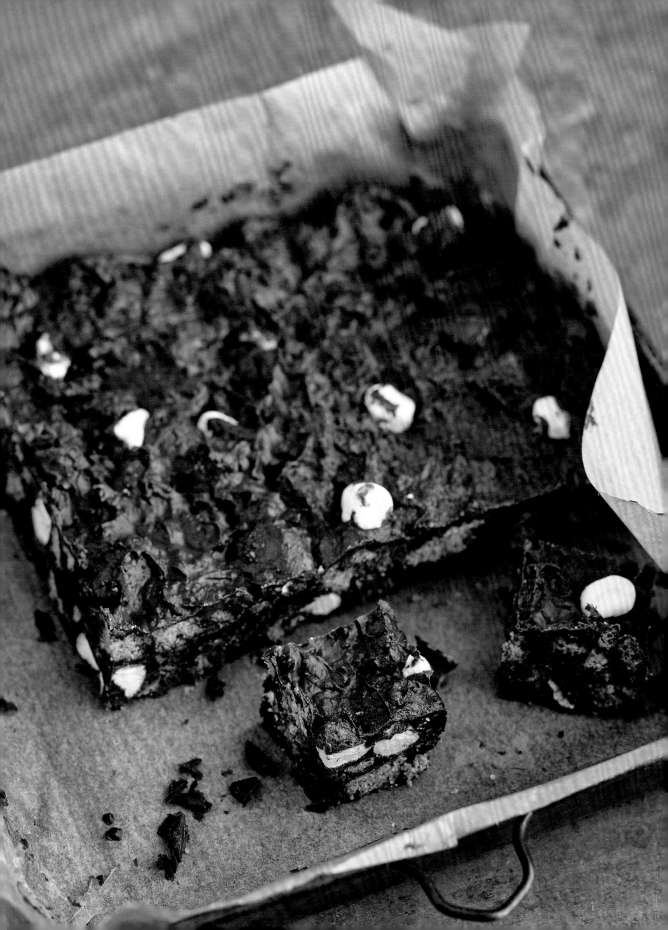

MAKES
15
SQUARES

PREP: 30 MINUTES,
PLUS CHILLING
COOK: 1 MINUTE

Warning: this cake is very hard to resist! Although it is made with dark chocolate, it is not bitter as the golden syrup and fruit make it lovely and sweet. This is very popular with Casper and his friends. We freeze it in ready-cut squares and find it useful to have batches in the freezer so that you can defrost one on the day of a party and take it along if your child can't have the cake being served. This recipe works particularly well using free-from ginger biscuits.

Rich Chocolate REFRIGERATOR CAKE

100g free-from
   biscuits
180g chocolate or
   dairy-free chocolate
   (70% cocoa solids),
   broken into pieces
50g golden syrup
45g dairy-free
   sunflower spread
30g raisins
50g glacé cherries, halved
Good handful mini
   marshmallows

1 Line a 15 x 20cm baking tray with greaseproof paper.

2 Break the biscuits up gently using a rolling pin – try not to make fine crumbs but aim to have little pieces.

3 Put the chocolate, golden syrup and sunflower spread in a microwave-safe bowl and heat in the microwave on high power for 10 seconds. Stir and repeat several times until the mixture is just melted and smooth.

4 Add the biscuit pieces, raisins, cherries and marshmallows to the chocolate mix and stir well.

5 Pour the mixture into the prepared tray and pop it in the fridge to cool, ideally overnight, before removing and cutting into squares with a sharp knife.

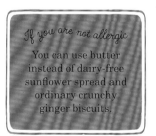

If you are not allergic
You can use butter instead of dairy-free sunflower spread and ordinary crunchy ginger biscuits.

MAKES 12 CAKES

PREP: 10 MINUTES,
PLUS CHILLING
COOK: 1 MINUTE

This is an old favourite that is a good alternative to cupcakes at parties. It is also great fun to get the kids involved making them as they are so easy to do. You can freeze them once they're set and like our Chocolate Refrigerator Cake (see page 225) and cupcakes (see page 210), it's handy having batches in the freezer so that you can take one out on the day of a party and take it along if your child can't have the cake being served. They also keep well in the fridge in a sealed container for up to three days.

Chocolate CRISPIE CAKES

100g dark chocolate
  (70% cocoa solids),
  broken into pieces ⬤
50g golden syrup
50g dairy-free
  sunflower spread
100g free-from breakfast
  cereal (rice crispie or
  cornflake style cereals
  are best) ⬤

Optional toppings
Dairy-free chocolate
  buttons ⬤
Mini marshmallows

1 Put the chocolate, golden syrup and sunflower spread in a microwave-safe bowl in the microwave. Heat for 10 seconds and then stir and repeat several times until the mixture is just melted and smooth.

2 Add the cereal and gently stir until it is all coated in the melted chocolate mixture.

3 Spoon the mixture into cupcake cases set out in a muffin tin or on a tray.

4 You can add toppings such as marshmallows or dairy-free chocolate buttons if you choose.

5 Pop in the fridge to set, ideally overnight.

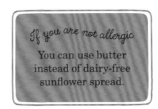

If you are not allergic
You can use butter
instead of dairy-free
sunflower spread.

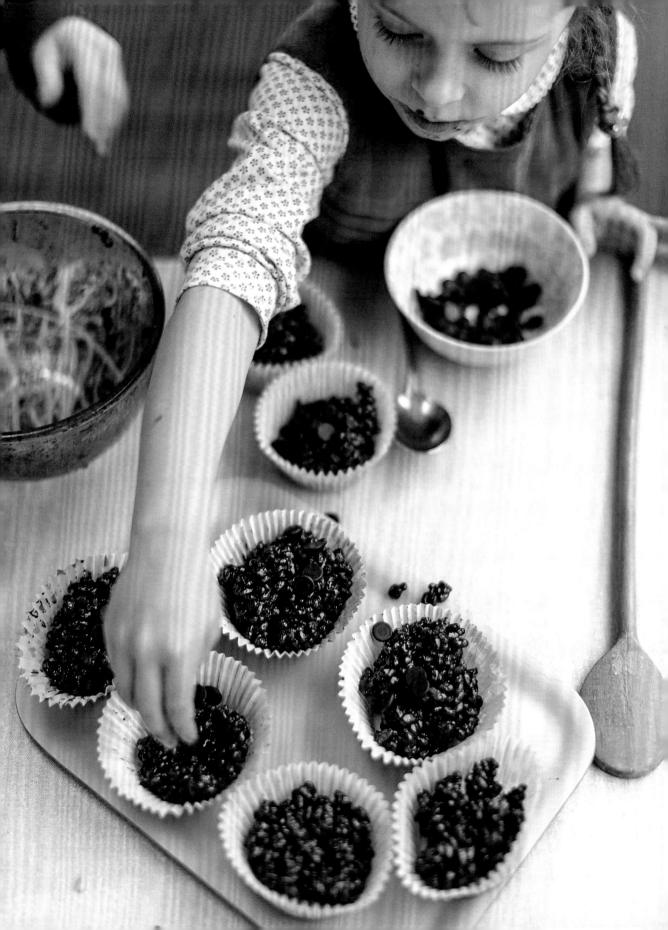

HOMEMADE JELLY

SERVES A FAMILY OF 4

PREP: 15 MINUTES,
PLUS CHILLING
COOK: 1 MINUTE

Most children love jelly and it is so easy to make your own. Our kids like apple and blackcurrant jelly. Cranberry, cherry and elderflower work very well for adults too. Avoid pineapple juice as it will not set in gelatine.

One-Colour Jelly

4 leaves gelatine
 (7x11cm)
320ml fruit juice
 of your choice
Fresh fruit (optional) –
 we like mandarin
 oranges, blueberries,
 raspberries, chopped
 strawberries and grapes

1 Pop the gelatine leaves in a bowl of cold water for 4 minutes. Remove the gelatine and shake off any excess water.

2 Place the gelatine in a small saucepan and set over a low heat for a few seconds until it has melted. Pour the fruit juice into the pan.

3 Stir until mixed well and then pour into individual bowls or glasses. Add any fruit you wish and then pop in the fridge to set for at least 2 hours.

Multi-Coloured Layered Jelly

3 x flavoured jelly
 (as above) or packet
 mixes – or as many
 colours/flavours as
 you wish to use

Our kids think it's really cool when we set jelly in multi-coloured layers. If you want to make a traffic light of green, amber and red you might wish to use packets of jelly as they have vibrant colours. However you wish to create your stripes remember to use a glass dish so they can be seen!

1 Mix up the jelly one colour at a time as you need it. (If using packets of jelly follow the instructions on the packet.)

2 Starting with the colour jelly you wish to have at the bottom, pour a little into each clear bowl or glass and pop in the fridge.

3 As soon as it starts to set (this will take up to an hour), add an equal layer of the next colour on top and pop back in the fridge.

4 Repeat with the next layer and so on until you are happy with your stripes.

5 Chill until all the jelly is set and serve.

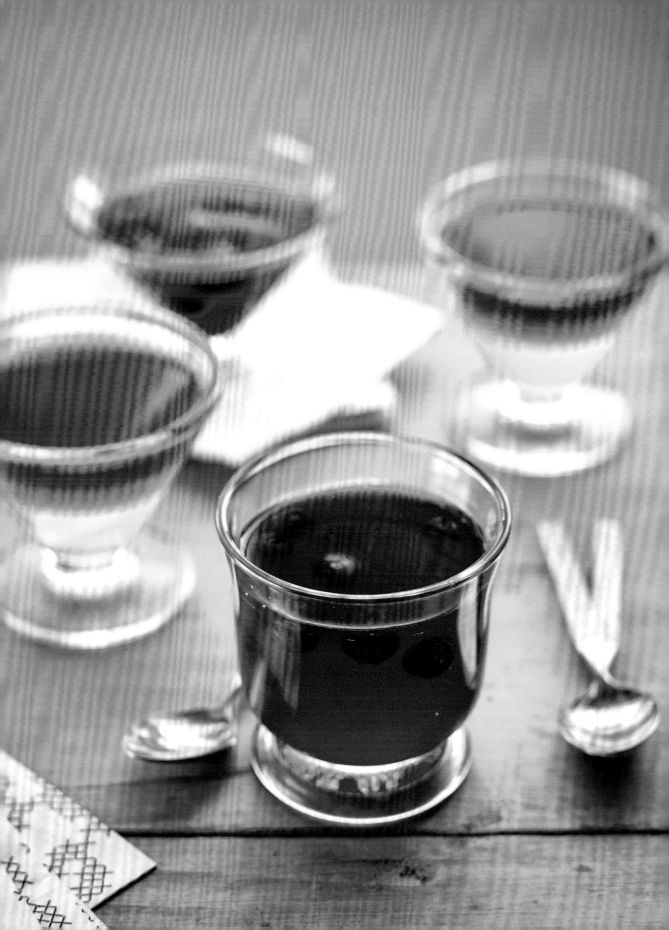

SERVES A FAMILY OF 4

PREP: 10 MINUTES
COOK: 1 MINUTE

This is a fun way to serve sliced fruit and kids (and grown-ups) love it – especially as it can be a little messy. If you have time, you can thread the fruit and marshmallows onto skewers to make fruit kebabs ready to be dipped in the chocolate.

Chocolate FONDUE

200g dairy-free chocolate
   buttons or dark
   chocolate (70%
   cocoa solids) ⚠
50g golden syrup
45g dairy-free
   sunflower spread
2 teaspoons water
Fresh fruit, such
   as strawberries,
   slices of orange,
   slices of banana,
   marshmallows
Long skewers

1 Put the chocolate, golden syrup and sunflower spread in a microwave-safe bowl and heat in a microwave for 10 seconds. Stir and repeat several times until the mixture is just melted and smooth.

2 Pour into individual ramekins and arrange the fruit around the ramekins with some skewers and serve.

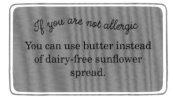

If you are not allergic
You can use butter instead of dairy-free sunflower spread.

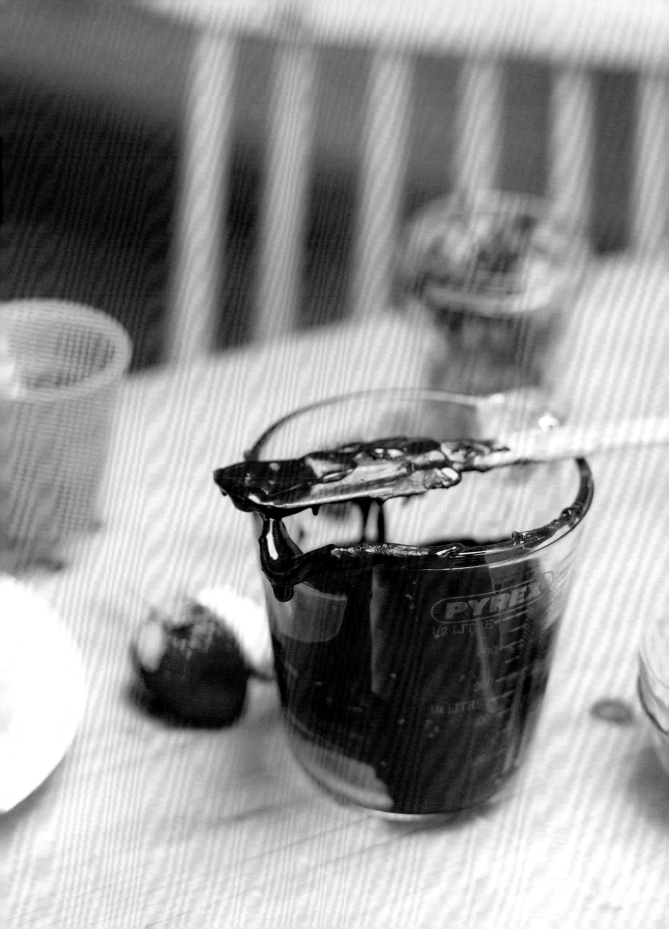

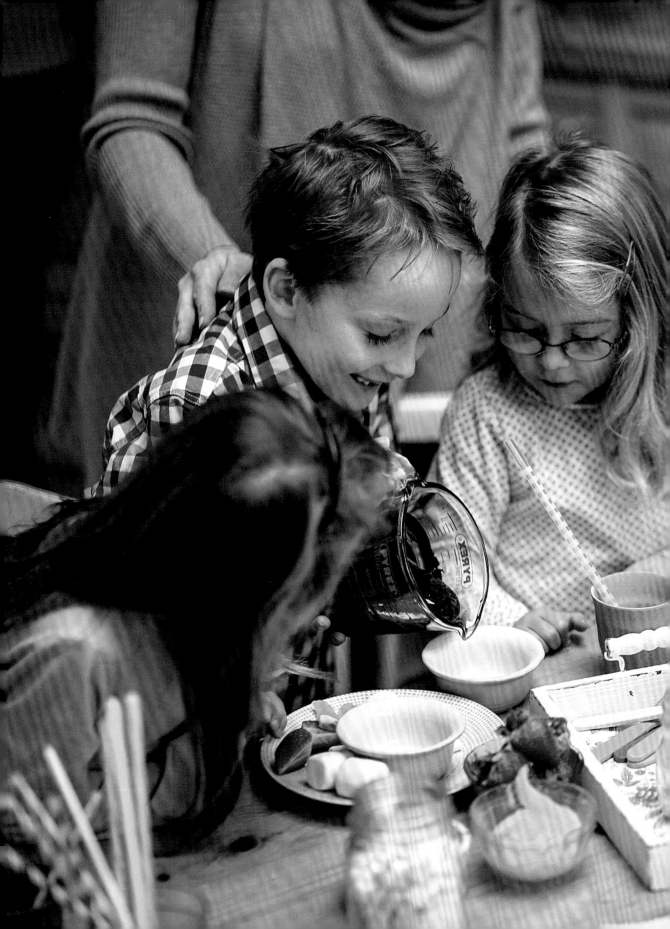

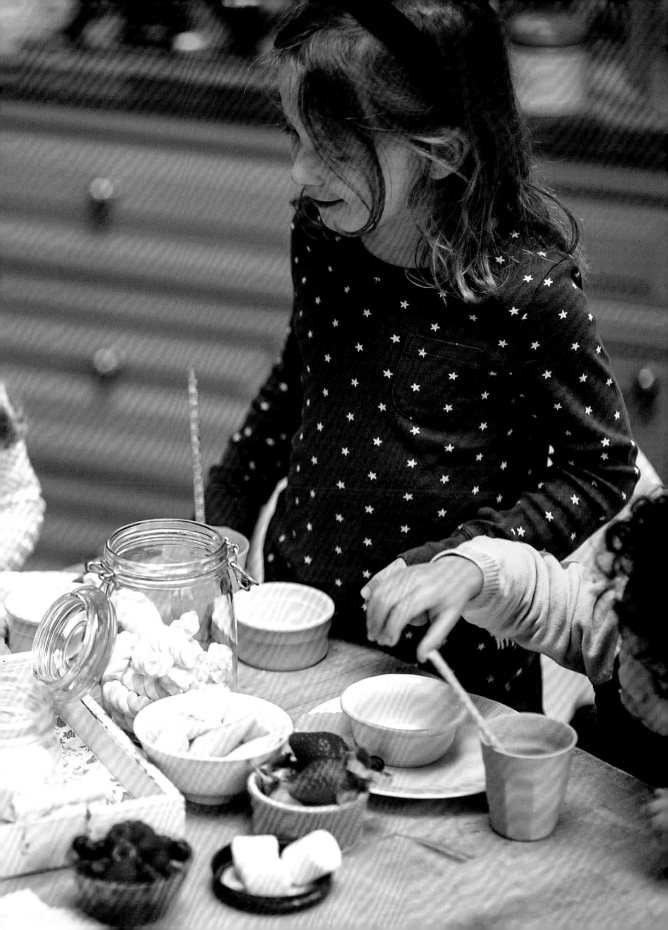

HOMEMADE ICE LOLLIES

MAKES 6 LOLLIES

PREP: 10 MINUTES,
PLUS FREEZING
COOK: NONE

Homemade lollies are easy to make and great because you know exactly what ingredients are in them so there's no need to worry about allergens or artificial additives or preservatives. The key to making fruit lollies is that the fruit must be really ripe, especially if you choose not to add any sugar. You will need lollipop moulds, which you can now buy from shops. All these lollies are best consumed within a week.

Orange, Mango and Coconut

1 small fresh mango,
 peeled and roughly
 chopped (about
 200g flesh)
Juice of 1 orange,
 freshly squeezed
1 teaspoon light or dark soft
 brown sugar (optional)
4 tablespoons coconut
 cream (not coconut milk)

Blend all the ingredients using a hand-held blender, adding sugar if you are using it.

Creamy Berry

2 good handfuls
 strawberries
2 good handfuls
 raspberries
Dash of orange juice
4 tablespoons
 coconut cream
 (not coconut milk)
1 teaspoon soft brown
 sugar (optional)

1 Blend the berries and juice using a hand-held blender. Pass through a sieve to remove all the seeds.

2 Return to the blender and add the coconut cream and sugar, if using.

3 Fill your tray of lolly moulds and freeze until set.

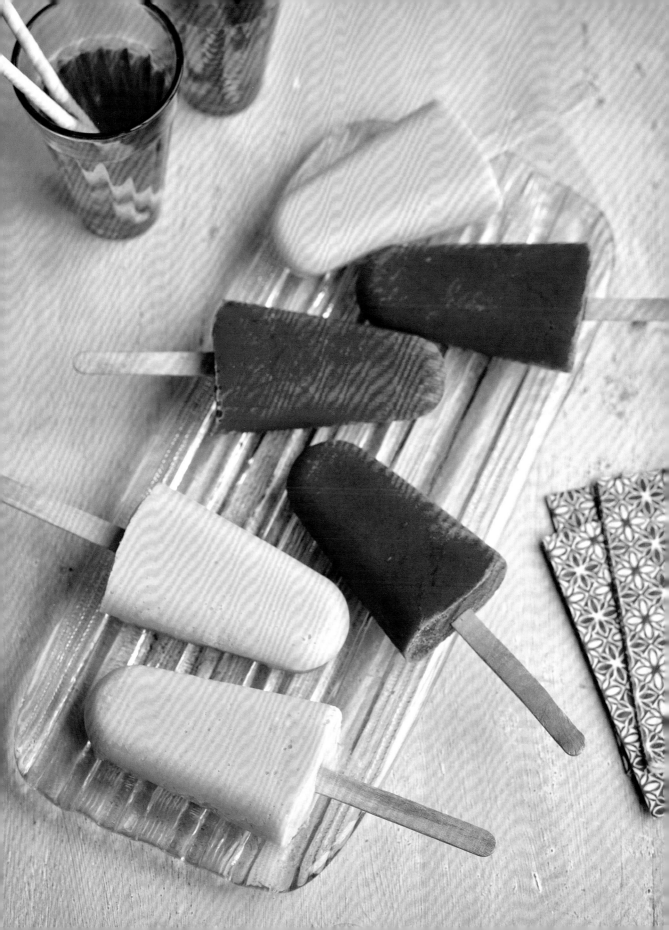

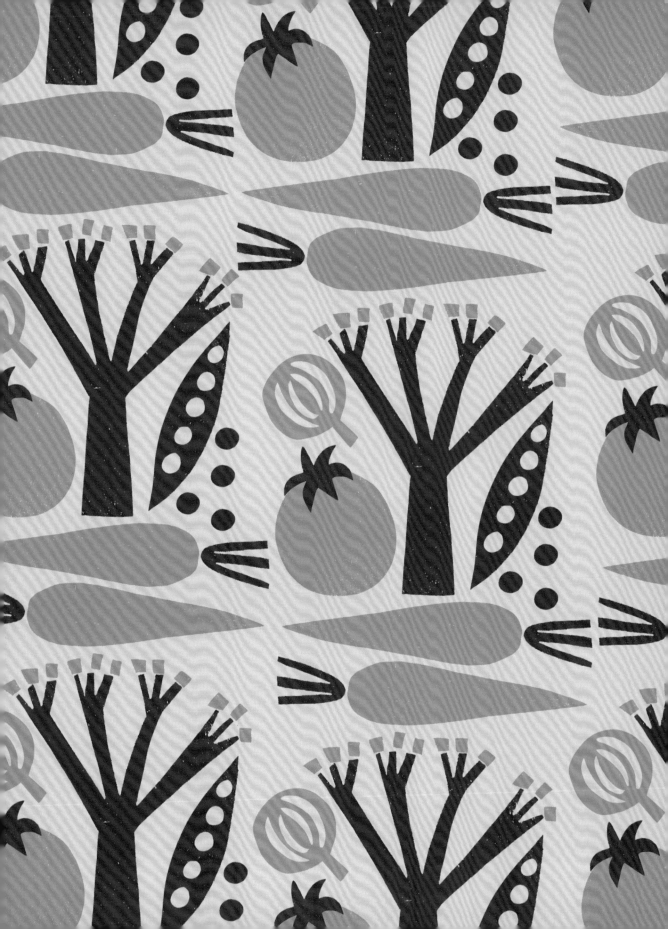

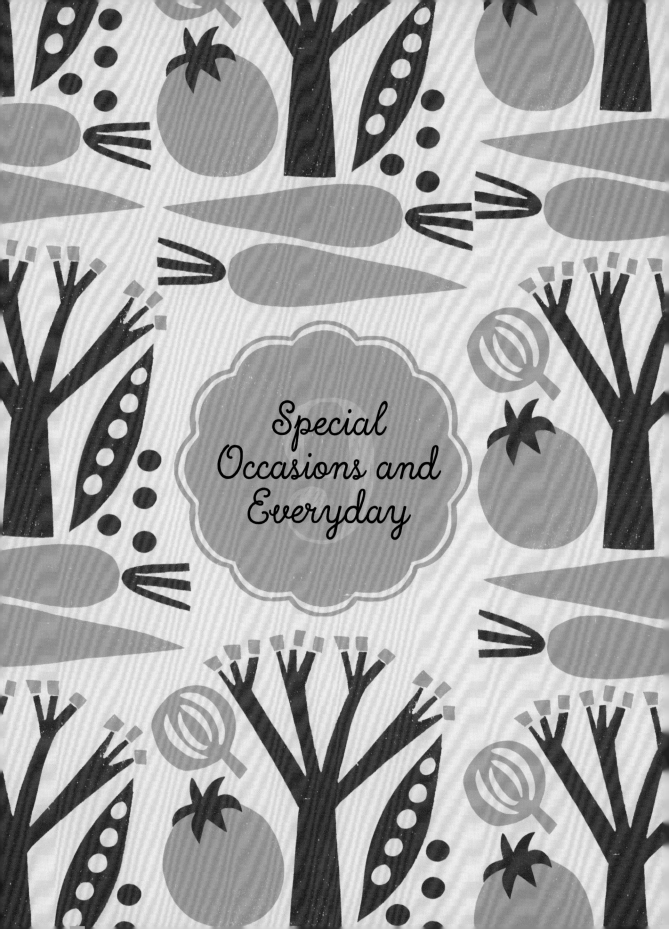

Special
Occasions and
Everyday

In this chapter we give you some ideas that we hope will help make it easier to plan for various events.

Our weekday mornings are always a bit of a manic rush to get everyone ready and out of the door on time. With finishing last-minute homework, brushing teeth, getting dressed, making hair presentable, packing school bags and the general morning mayhem, you want breakfast to be effortless. Toast and cereal are breakfast staples but not an option for dairy, soya and gluten allergy sufferers unless you buy free-from options of which there is an increasing, but still limited, choice. If you want a bit more variety, we've given you a range of suggestions to make breakfast more interesting without making your morning routine more frantic.

Making a packed lunch every day can seem like a chore – yet another thing to do in the morning – and it's harder when easy options like sandwiches are off the menu unless you use free-from products. You can make really wholesome packed lunches every day without racking your brains by using our suggested options in this chapter.

We've been to lots of barbecues and picnics and they can often be a bit of a headache even when there is food our children can eat. Normally there is a big spread with lots of bowls of different salads and sides but often people don't think twice about using the same spoon in different bowls and food can easily drop from one bowl to another as guests help themselves, resulting in cross contamination of allergens. We find the best solution is to bring your child's own food but it's even nicer if you're hosting an event to make all the food allergy free and then there's no risk of cross contamination of allergens. We think our food is so good that your guests without food allergy will be none the wiser.

Birthday parties are always great fun and our children really look forward to theirs months and months beforehand. You can make almost any shaped cake using our basic chocolate cake recipe (see page 210) and ice it however you like. We suggest lots of party food ideas in this chapter that have always gone down well with all the kids at the parties we've organised for our own children.

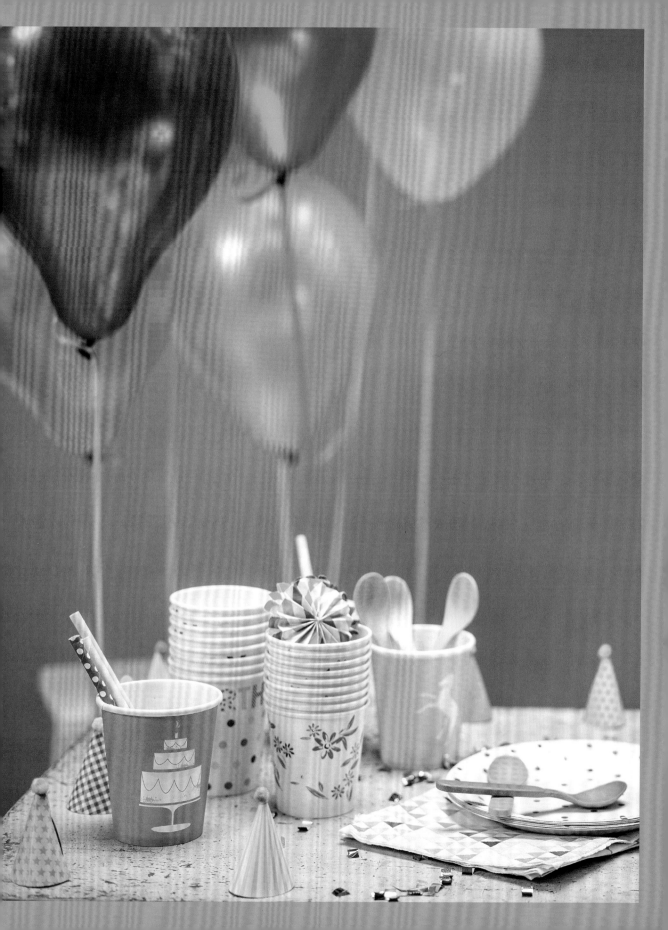

PACKED LUNCH IDEAS

Packed lunches can be really easy when you have a child with allergies especially if you are organised. It's a good idea to have different-sized airtight plastic tubs to hand to pop food in. By using tubs you can keep the food fresh and individual to your child so you can make sure there is no cross contamination of ingredients or other people's food.

All of these options can be made the night before your picnic or school run. Just prepare them, then chill in the fridge ready to go the next day. If you pop a small ice brick in the bag, or a frozen drink, it can help keep things cold.

Sandwiches (using gluten-free and egg-free bread and dairy-free spread) are probably the most basic staple in a packed lunch and you can use meat from a leftover roast as a healthier alternative to ham or processed meat. If you only need to make the occasional packed lunch you may want to be a bit more elaborate than if you are making a daily packed lunch but the ideas below also provide a little variety if your child is having a packed lunch every day.

FILLING YOUR LUNCHBOX

Recipes that make great lunchbox fillers:

* Baby New Potato Salad (see page 180)
* Three Bean Salad (see page 142)
* Eggless Niçoise Salad (see page 78) just tear the lettuce leaves up small enough so they are easy to pop in the tub and eat with a fork
* Rice Salad (see page 143)
* Cold Chicken Kebabs (see page 87)
* Vegetable crudités and Hummus (see page 132)
* Carrot with Poppy Seeds (see page 140)
* Pasta Salad (see page 145)
* Puy Lentil Salad (see page 148)
* Quinoa Salad (see page 150)
* Coleslaw (see page 146)
* Jam Tarts (see page 213) – no need to chill these
* Jelly (see page 228) – set the jelly in the tub
* Sushi (see page 198)

SOME OTHER EASY OPTIONS:

* Pieces of fruit – peel and/or chop at home so they are ready to eat
* Packet of rice cakes or corn crackers !
* Packet of crisps !
* Free-from biscuits !
* Cold sausages !
* Cold leftover pieces of roast chicken, beef or lamb
* Cold piece of poached salmon
* Fruit pots or pouches

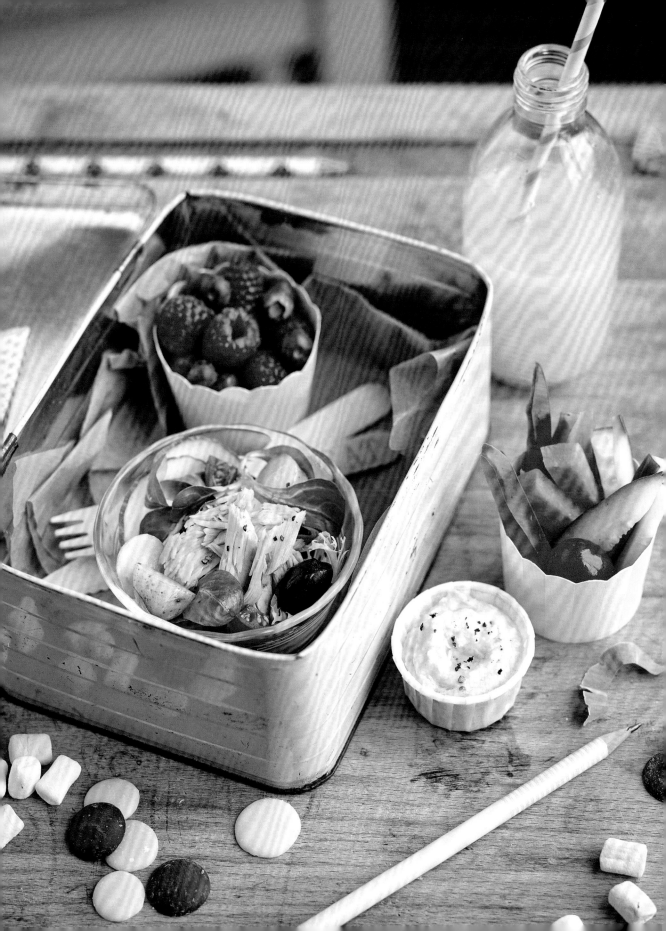

BREAKFAST IDEAS

Breakfast is such an important meal. We all really want to set our kids up for a good day with a nice full tummy and having allergies does limit a traditional breakfast as gluten and dairy items feature highly on the menu. There are some great free-from alternatives in the supermarket such as cereals, breads and milks but here is a list of suggestions and pointers to recipes you can find elsewhere in this book to help you keep breakfast interesting for your children, especially for those who can't have dairy or gluten.

Don't worry if you think what you might be serving your child is not a traditional breakfast – the most important thing is they have something nutritious inside them to set them up for the day, so if on some days you find yourself cooking a plate of gluten-free pasta and sauce for breakfast, don't worry!

BREAKFAST SAVIOURS

* Fruit Smoothies (see page 206)
* Grapefruit segments
* Pan-fried leftover potatoes or Bubble and Squeak (see page 161)
* Grilled bacon
* Sausages !
* Baked beans on potato waffles !
* Poached fish and rice
* Fruit Salad (see page 219)
* Cucumber sticks with Hummus (see page 132)
* Free-from fish fingers
* Garlic mushrooms with Lemon and Parsley (see page 156)

BIRTHDAY PARTIES

Birthday parties are such a special part of growing up. You don't want your child to miss out because of a food allergy and there's no reason why they should. Children always so look forward to their birthday party and it doesn't need to be a nightmare for you. If you're hosting your child's party you can have complete control of the menu, which makes things a bit easier. In reality, none of the kids at the party will realise they are eating food that is free from allergens as it is all standard party fare and your child can enjoy everything at the party with all their friends. It's good to prepare everything at home and then transport it to the venue.

ESSENTIAL PARTY FOOD

Here are some party food ideas that all children will enjoy – those with and without food allergies.

* Honey-glazed sausages on sticks (see below) !
* Finger sandwiches (with a variety of fillings such as ham, jam, cucumber) on gluten- and egg-free bread !
* Hot or cold chicken skewers or strips if you have young children (see page 87)
* Cucumber and smoked salmon Sushi (see page 198)
* Cocktail sausages with tomato ketchup dip (see below)
* Cherry tomatoes
* Cucumber, carrot, red and yellow pepper, crudités with Hummus (see page 132) and Guacamole (see page 133)
* Crisps !
* Strawberries and berries
* Slices of watermelon
* Multi-Coloured Layered Jelly (see page 228)
* Chocolate Refrigerator Cake (see page 225)
* Chocolate Crispie Cakes (see page 226)
* Chocolate characters (see below)
* Birthday cake (see below and page 210)

HONEY-GLAZED SAUSAGES ON STICKS

Buy chipolata sausages that are allergen-free. Cut each sausage into three and roast in the oven until cooked. Halfway through cooking add a good drizzle of honey. Once cooked arrange on the plate and put a cocktail stick in each one (for smaller children it's probably safer without the cocktail sticks). Alternatively, you could leave out the honey and serve with a little dish of tomato ketchup for dipping.

With all sausages, leave to cool sufficiently before serving to children, or chill and serve cold.

CHOCOLATE CHARACTERS

Simply melt some suitable dairy-free chocolate in the microwave, 10 seconds at a time until just melted and then spoon carefully into silicone ice trays. There are lots of ice trays in shops with kids' favourite characters from Lego mini-figures to Hello Kitty. Chill in the fridge and when set, turn out of the moulds. Please note that if you don't use silicone trays you may have trouble getting the shapes out!

BIRTHDAY CAKE

Our Really Chocolately Chocolate Cake is a huge hit with kids and grown-ups with and without allergies. It is the perfect birthday cake and can easily be iced to suit your theme. Use our chocolate icing detailed in the recipe or buy ready-to-roll icing in any colour to suit your party. Ellie has successfully used the cake to make a princess and it looked and tasted fabulous. See page 210 for the recipe.

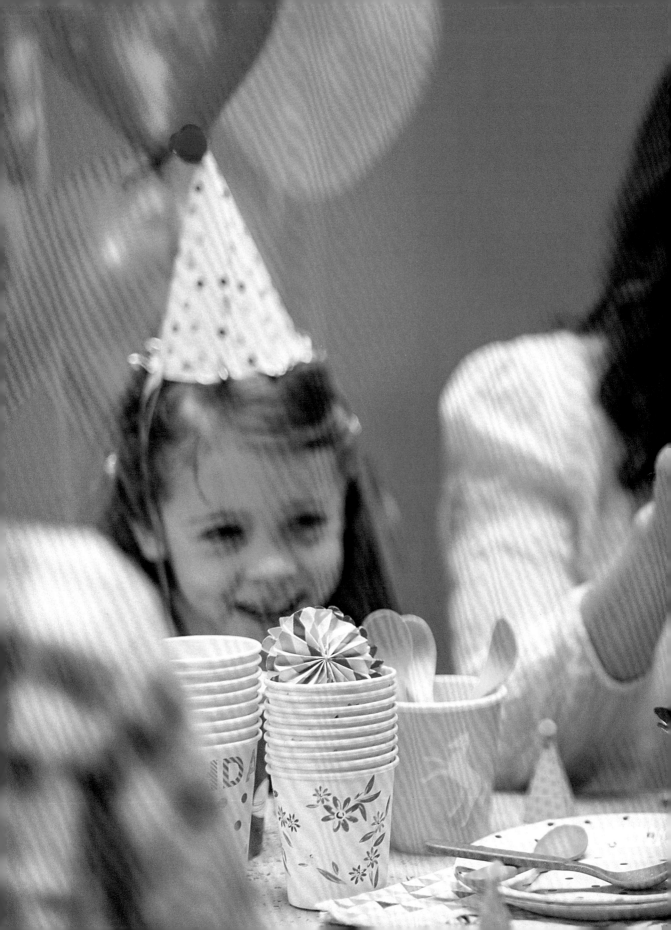

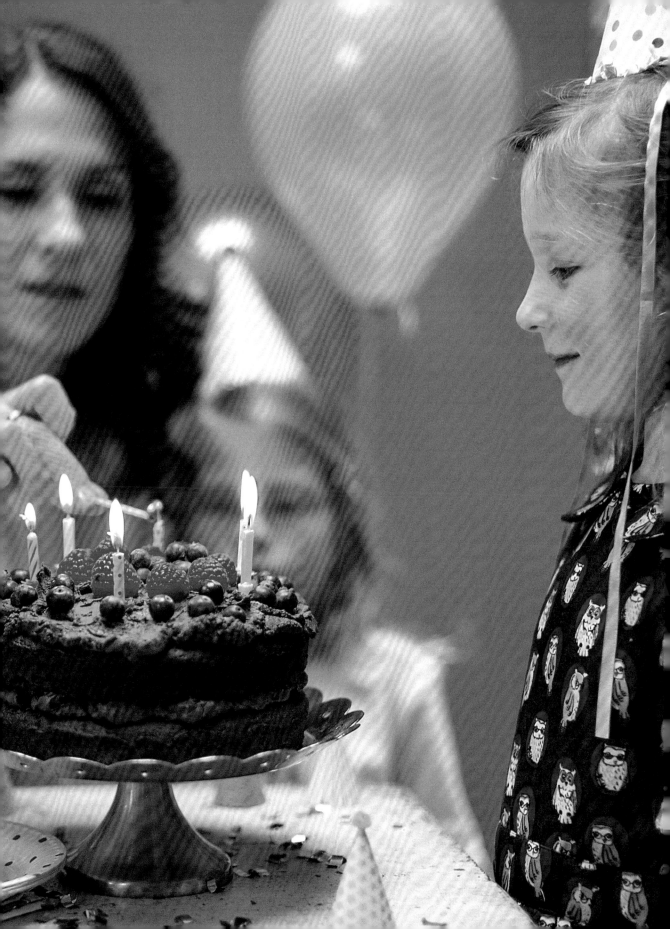

It is really useful to have a couple of basic stock recipes if you want to avoid manufactured stocks, which can be high in salt and often contain allergens such as egg, flour and celery. Stocks are very easy to make and are a good way to use a leftover chicken after a roast or leftover vegetables. The key to making a good stock is to allow it to simmer very gently on your hob for a long time. This will give you a lovely clear stock with tons of flavour.

Our Homemade Southeast Asian Blend (see page 251) is a combination of herbs and spices including coriander and lemongrass that forms the base for a number of recipes in this book. It is worth making in a large batch and putting it in the freezer so you always have some to hand and don't need to do lots of chopping each time you make one of our Southeast Asian recipes such as Vietnamese Rice Noodle Soup (see page 81) or Mild Thai Coconut Chicken Curry (see page 48). This makes them very quick to prepare.

Our classic gravy recipe goes well with most roasts and is of course free from allergens commonly found in gravy, such as gluten.

10

Easy Stocks and Essentials

MAKES ABOUT 1L

PREP: 5 MINUTES
COOK: 40 MINUTES

Vegetable stock can be used in lots of recipes to give more flavour to the meal you are cooking. It really is very simple and worth trying especially if you have never made stock before. Make ahead of time, cool and keep in the fridge for up to one week. Or reduce further and freeze, just remembering to dilute again when using in recipes.

Simple VEGETABLE STOCK

2 tablespoons olive oil
1 large onion, chopped
  into chunks with
  skin left on
1 carrot, chopped
2 celery sticks, chopped
  (optional)
2 garlic cloves, crushed
A few fresh parsley stems
4 black peppercorns
1 bay leaf
2 litres water

1 Heat the oil in a large heavy-based pan over a medium heat and then cook the onion, carrot and celery for about 5 minutes, allowing them to soften.

2 Add the garlic, parsley, peppercorns, bay leaf and water and bring to the boil.

3 Reduce the heat and simmer very gently for about 30 minutes, skimming off any scum and fat as necessary.

4 Strain off the liquid into a pan and discard the vegetables. Reduce further if necessary.

If you are not allergic
Use the optional celery

SERVES A FAMILY OF 4

PREP: 5 MINUTES
COOK: 5 MINUTES

This is a real must when you have a roast dinner and very easy to do. It is essentially the lovely pan juices thickened with some cornflour.

Easy GRAVY

Pan juices from
   roasted meat
2 teaspoons cornflour
1 tablespoon cold water
100–300ml fresh stock
   (see pages 248 and 250)
   or the liquid from your
   boiled or steamed
   vegetables if cooking
   at the same time

1 Remove the meat from your roasting tin and skim off any excess fat. It is important to leave about a tablespoon of fat in the pan as it helps with flavour. Pop the roasting tin on the hob over a medium heat and stir well, making sure you have scraped all the lovely cooked bits from the sides and bottom of the pan.

2 Mix the cornflour and cold water in a separate bowl and stir well, then tip it straight into the roasting pan and mix really well.

3 Bring to a gentle simmer, stirring continually and you will see all the juices start to thicken into a lovely gravy.

4 Add the stock or vegetable cooking liquid to the gravy, adjusting the amount to your desired consistency.

VARIATION
If you wish you can make onion gravy by adding 1 peeled and sliced onion in the first stage and allowing the onion to soften and cook for about 10 minutes before you add the cornflour and follow the rest of the recipe. If you prefer gravy with a darker colour, simply cook the onions on a higher heat to allow them to caramelise but not burn before following the rest of the recipe.

MAKES ABOUT 500 ML

PREP: 5 MINUTES
COOK: 1¼ HOURS

This is easy to make after a roast chicken – don't waste the leftover bones! This stock is the basis for several recipes and is easy to freeze. Simply reduce further to concentrate the stock and freeze, remembering to dilute again when using in recipes. You can freeze the stock in an ice-cube tray and once frozen the cubes can be placed inside a freezer bag so that you can use them as and when you need them.

White CHICKEN STOCK

1 chicken carcass
1 onion, chopped
1 carrot, chopped
2 celery sticks, chopped (optional)
A few fresh parsley stems
4 black peppercorns
1 bay leaf
2 litres of water

If you are not allergic
Use the optional celery

1 Put all the ingredients in a large heavy-based pan and then very slowly bring to the boil.

2 As soon as it boils, reduce the heat and simmer very gently for about 1 hour. It is the very low simmer that will give the best results and flavour – don't be tempted to boil it to speed up the cooking process – you will end up with a cloudy, fatty stock. Skim off any scum and fat as necessary.

3 Strain the liquid into a bowl and discard the bones and vegetables.

4 Reduce further to about 500ml of liquid.

MAKES
4
TABLESPOONS

PREP: 10 MINUTES
COOK: NONE

This aromatic blend of herbs and spices is a basis for our Southeast Asian inspired recipes such as our Vietnamese Rice Noodle Soup (see page 81), Mild Thai Chicken Coconut Curry (see page 48) and our Mild Fish Curry (see page 102). As most of these herbs come pre-packed or bundled, don't waste any, just increase the recipe to suit the quantities that you have so there are no leftovers. Freeze in a tub or ziplock bag so it is easy to take a spoonful whenever you need some.

Homemade SOUTHEAST ASIAN BLEND

4 teaspoons finely chopped shallots

2 teaspoons peeled and finely chopped fresh ginger

2 teaspoons chopped fresh coriander leaves and stems

2 teaspoons finely chopped lemongrass stems

1 teaspoon crushed garlic

1 teaspoon finely chopped kaffir lime leaves (remove the woody stem before chopping)

¼ teaspoon chopped red chilli (optional – only if you want some heat)

Mix all the ingredients together in a bowl and then either use immediately or freeze for another time.

INDEX

FURTHER INFORMATION

The first place to get advice about your child's allergy should always be your doctor and dietitian but if you want to do a bit more research yourself there are lots of charities with very helpful websites. Websites change and new ones pop up, but at the time of writing these were all correct.

WWW.ACTIONAGAINSTALLERGY.CO.UK

WWW.ALLERGYUK.ORG

WWW.ANAPHYLAXIS.ORG.UK

WWW.ASTHMA.ORG.UK

WWW.COELIAC.ORG.UK

WWW.ECZEMA.ORG

WWW.EFANET.ORG

WWW.FABED.CO.UK

WWW.FOOD.GOV.UK

WWW.FOODSMATTER.COM

WWW.NHS.UK

WWW.PARENTSOWN.CO.UK

DIRECTORY OF READY-MADE FREE-FROM FOODS AND ESSENTIAL INGREDIENTS

Please have a look at our website www.foodallergymums.co.uk where we list all our children's favourite ready-made, free-from foods. From bread, pasta and flour to biscuits, chocolate and puddings to spreads, mayonnaise and sauces we've compiled a comprehensive list of delicious free-from foods and basic ingredients that will help make life a little easier and supplement your home-cooked meals. It's surprising how many good products there are out there that suit almost any combination of food allergies.

Follow us on Twitter 🐦 @foodallergymums

ACKNOWLEDGEMENTS

Isabelle and Casper introduced us to the world of food allergy and were the inspiration for this book. They, along with their sisters Zara and Camille, have eaten all the recipes in this book (plus quite a few which didn't make the grade). They were all brutally honest and never held back if they decided something wasn't up to scratch.

We would like to thank Dr Helen Cox, a leading paediatric allergy and immunology consultant, and Dr Rosan Meyer, a dietitian at the top of her field, for all their energy and input in making sure that this book is useful and informative and most importantly accurate from a medical perspective. They were extremely generous with their time, making sure the content of this book is sound and the recipes are nutritious and allergen-free. Given that they hold several busy clinics and lecture all over the world this was a very valuable gift.

Dr Cox has written a wonderful foreword to this book, answering many questions that parents of children with food allergy would like answered but may not remember to ask during a doctor's appointment.

We would also like to thank Zoe Cordy-Simpson, freelance recipe tester, and her daughter, Rose, who tested a number of recipes in the book.

Jenny Stringer, Fiona's principal at Leith's, has been a wonderful source of guidance and help. Additional thanks must go to Alison Cavaliero. Fiona would like to especially thank Gary Rhodes who she met at one of his book signings. He generously offered her a day's work experience at City Rhodes, his busy London restaurant. This led to a career change into the exciting world of food and she's never looked back.

Amanda Harris at Orion has been fantastic: she really understood our concept and has brought it to life in a way we couldn't have imagined. The whole team at Orion couldn't have been more supportive or helpful throughout the publication process. We would particularly like to thank our wonderfully patient editors Tamsin English, Abi Waters and Kate Wanwimolruk. Chris Terry, our photographer, brought a wealth of experience and good humour (especially photographing the children) and we are thrilled with the results. Thanks must also go to Helen Ewing, Smith & Gilmour, Olivia Wardle and Henrietta Clancy for providing their creative and artistic flair to make this such a beautiful book.

Our agent, Clare Hulton, has given us lots of guidance and has been a pleasure to work with throughout.

Most importantly we are hugely grateful to our husbands, Ben Wright and Matt Katz, for their positive encouragement and support. Along with our children and good friends, they have given us valuable feedback ensuring all our recipes are delicious for everyone regardless of food allergy.